The Natural Medicine Guide to

ANXIETY

Also by Stephanie Marohn

Natural Medicine First Aid Remedies

Other Titles in the ***Healthy Mind Guide*** Series:

The Natural Medicine Guide to Autism

The Natural Medicine Guide to Depression

The Natural Medicine Guide to Bipolar Disorder

The Natural Medicine Guide to Schizophrenia

THE HEALTHY MIND GUIDES

The Natural Medicine Guide to

ANXIETY

Stephanie Marohn

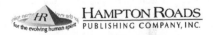

HAMPTON ROADS
PUBLISHING COMPANY, INC.

Cover design by Bookwrights Design
Cover art/photographic image © 2003 Loyd Chapplow

Hampton Roads Publishing Company, Inc.
1125 Stoney Ridge Road
Charlottesville, VA 22902

434-296-2772
fax: 434-296-5096
e-mail: hrpc@hrpub.com
www.hrpub.com

If you are unable to order this book from your local
bookseller, you may order directly from the publisher.
Call 1-800-766-8009, toll-free.

Library of Congress Cataloging-in-Publication Data

Marohn, Stephanie.
  The natural medicine guide to anxiety / Stephanie Marohn.
     p. cm. -- (Healthy mind guides)
Includes bibliographical references and index.
  ISBN 1-57174-293-X
  1. Anxiety--Alternative treatment. 2. Naturopathy. I. Title. II.
Series.
  RC537.M3728 2003
  616.85'22306--dc22

                                    2003021693

ISBN 1-57174-293-X
10 9 8 7 6 5 4 3 2 1
Printed on acid-free paper in Canada

THE HEALTHY 🙘 MIND GUIDES

The Healthy Mind Guides are a series of books offering original research and treatment options for reversing or ameliorating so-called mental disorders, written by noted health journalist and author Stephanie Marohn. The series' focus is the natural medicine approach, a refreshing and hopeful outlook based on treating individual needs rather than medical labels, and addressing the underlying imbalances—biological, psychological, emotional, and spiritual.

Each book in the series offers the very latest information about the possible causes of each disorder, and presents a wide range of effective, practical therapies drawn from extensive interviews with physicians and other practitioners who are innovators in their respective fields. Case studies throughout the books illustrate the applications of these therapies, and numerous resources are provided for readers who want to seek treatment.

ى

To the end of the reign of fear

Contents

Acknowledgments

My deep gratitude to all of the following:

The doctors and other healing professionals who shared information on their work for this book:

Ira J. Golchehreh, L.Ac., O.M.D.
Patricia Kaminski
Dietrich Klinghardt, M.D., Ph.D.
Carola M. Lage-Roy
Reverend Leon S. LeGant
Thomas M. Rau, M.D.
Judyth Reichenberg-Ullman, N.D., L.C.S.W.
Tony Roffers, Ph.D.
Malidoma Patrice Somé, Ph.D.
Zannah Steiner, C.M.P., R.M.T.

Nan and Bob Marohn for generous patronage of the arts
The Gaia Circle and Ballet Maestra Nancy Gallenson for
providing antidotes to anxiety
Sue Trowbridge and Dorothy Anderson for transcribing
many interviews
Donna Canali, Mella Mincberg, and Moli Steinert for our
precious friendship and your many-mansioned support
Richard Leviton for dogged determination, wit, and vision

Introduction

While depression and Prozac have become household words in the United States, prompting some to dub our times "the age of melancholy," it is equally true that we are living in "the age of anxiety." The incidence of anxiety disorders rose dramatically in the second half of the twentieth century, to the point that they are now the most common "mental" illness.[1] According to the World Health Organization, the odds of developing an anxiety disorder are double what they were 40 years ago.[2] In a given year, one in nine Americans are now suffering from an anxiety disorder.[3] One in four people will be afflicted in the course of their lifetime.[4]

The twin epidemics of anxiety and depression are part of the massive mental health crisis currently facing the United States and other countries in the developed world. The psychiatric treatment methods we have been using are not working, as is clear from the dire statistics on mental illness. Here are just a few of the startling facts:

- Mental illness is the second leading cause of disability and premature mortality in the U.S. and other developed countries.[5]

- 4 of the 10 leading causes of disability in the U.S. and other developed countries are mental disorders—obsessive-compulsive disorder (an anxiety disorder), major depression, bipolar disorder, or schizophrenia.[6]

- 5.4% of adults in the U.S. have a serious mental illness (defined as "substantial interference with one or more major life activities"; less severe mental illness is not included in this statistic).[7]

- 1 in 4 hospital admissions in the U.S. in 1998 were psychiatric admissions.[8]

- $148 billion = the total cost of mental health services in the U.S. in 1990[9] ($69 billion in direct costs for mental health treatment and rehabilitation, and $79 billion in the indirect costs of lost productivity at work, school, or home due to disability or death).

A large reason why treatment of mental illness has a poor success record and is costing more all the time is because the overwhelming emphasis is placed on pharmaceutical drugs. Not everyone in the psychiatric field is happy with the ever-increasing governance of psychopharmacology (the science of drugs used to affect behavior and emotional states). Here is what one psychiatrist had to say about it. In December 1998, in a letter of resignation to the president of the American Psychiatric Association (APA), Loren R. Mosher, M.D., former official of the National Institute of Mental Health (NIMH), wrote:[10]

> After nearly three decades as a member it is with a mixture of pleasure and disappointment that I submit this letter of resignation from the American Psychiatric Association. The major reason for this action is my belief that I am actually resigning from the American Psychopharmacological Association. . . . At this point in history, in my view, psychiatry has been almost completely bought out by the drug companies. . . . We condone and promote the widespread overuse and misuse of toxic chemicals that we know have serious long term effects. . . .

While psychiatric drugs (prescription drugs used for mental illnesses) may control certain disorders, and in some instances save lives, they do not cure the disorder, and they often compound the person's problems with disturbing side effects in the short term and the risk of permanent damage in the long term. If we are going to solve the current mental health crisis, we are going to have to turn to other approaches to treatment.

The state of affairs in psychiatric treatment is reflected in the focus of quite a few of the books on mental illness aimed at the general public. The help they offer involves information for the patient on managing symptoms and coping with hospitalization; for family members on how to live with the disorder in a loved one; and on how to work with side effects of anxiolytics (antianxiety drugs), antidepressants, and other psychopharmaceuticals (psychiatric drugs), that is, what other drugs you can take to reduce those effects.

There are a number of useful books covering a range of anxiety-management methods, such as cognitive-behavioral therapy (CBT), exposure therapy, visualization, guided imagery, meditation, relaxation techniques, and breathing exercises. While these coping methods can be important and quite effective, they don't address the underlying causes of anxiety, except when psychological/emotional causes emerge during the therapy or practice.

For this reason and because there is plenty of good information on these techniques, I do not cover them in *The Natural Medicine Guide to Anxiety.* This book is dedicated to

This book is dedicated to exploring the underlying causes of anxiety, with the goal of healing from an anxiety disorder, rather than learning to live with it. To this end, the book offers a range of treatment approaches to address the causes and truly restore health.

exploring the underlying causes of anxiety, with the goal of healing from an anxiety disorder, rather than learning to live with it. To this end, the book offers a range of treatment approaches to address the causes and truly restore health.

Only by treating the underlying causes of anxiety, rather than suppressing the symptoms as drugs do, can lasting recovery be achieved. And only by considering the well-being of the mind and spirit as well as the body can comprehensive healing take place.

All of the therapies covered here approach the treatment of anxiety in this way. They all also share the characteristic of tailoring treatment to the individual, which is another essential element for a successful outcome. No two people, even with the same diagnosis, have exactly the same imbalances causing their problems.

With the increase in the number of people who are using natural therapies, the public has become more aware of this medical approach. When many people think of natural medicine, however, they think of supplements or herbal remedies available over the counter. While these products can be highly beneficial, natural medicine is far more than that. Natural therapies are those that operate according to holistic principles, meaning treating the whole person rather than an isolated part or symptom and using natural treatments that "Do no harm" and support or restore the body's natural ability to heal itself.

Natural medicine involves a way of looking at healing that is dramatically different from the conventional medical model. It does not mimic that model by merely substituting the herbal medicine kava-kava for an anxiolytic or St. John's wort for an antidepressant. Instead, it is the comprehensive approach described above, which offers you the possibility of curing your anxiety disorder.

That said, as with the anxiety-management techniques cited above, herbal and other natural remedies can be a useful corollary in alleviating your anxiety while you explore the deeper causes. Again, as there is already ample information on this subject and it doesn't fit with the in-depth treatment focus of this book, I don't cover it here. (For self-help treatments for anxiety, see my book *Natural Medicine First Aid Remedies*, Hampton Roads, 2001.)

Before I tell you a little about what's in this book, I would just like to say a few words about the terms "mental illness" and "mental disorders"—or "brain disorders" as they are more currently labeled. All of these terms reflect the disconnection between body and mind—never mind spirit—in conventional medical treatment. The newer term, brain disorders, reflects the biochemical model of causality that currently dominates the medical profession.

I use the terms "mental illness" and "mental disorders" in this book because there is no easy substitute that reflects the true body-mind-spirit nature of these conditions. While I may use these terms, I in no way mean to suggest that the causes of the disorders lie solely in the mind. The same is true for the title of the series of which this book is a part: *The Healthy Mind Guides*. The name serves to distinguish the subject area, but it is healthy mind, body, and spirit—wholeness—that is the focus of these books.

While I'm at it, I may as well dispense with one last linguistic issue. As natural medicine effects profound healing, rather than simply controlling symptoms, I prefer the term "natural medicine" over "alternative medicine." This medical model is not "other"—it is a primary form of medicine. The term "holistic medicine" reflects this as well, in that it signals the natural medicine approach of treating the whole person, rather than the parts.

Part 1 of *The Natural Medicine Guide to Anxiety* covers the basics of anxiety: what it is, who gets it, and what causes it. The natural medicine view is that many different factors (physical, psychological, and spiritual), often in combination, produce anxiety.

Part 2 of the book covers a range of natural medicine treatments for anxiety. The material presented here is based on research and interviews with physicians and other healing professionals who are leaders and pioneers in their respective fields. This is original information, not derivative material gleaned from secondary sources. The therapeutic techniques of these highly skilled doctors and other healers are explained in detail and illustrated with case studies that give a human face to anxiety and demonstrate the effectiveness of the therapies. (The names of patients throughout the book have been changed. Contact information for the practitioners whose work is presented appears in appendix B: Resources.)

To begin part 2, chapter 3 presents a model of healing that delineates the five levels of a person that must be restored to balance if complete health and well-being are to be achieved. The five levels—Physical, Electromagnetic, Mental, Intuitive, and Spiritual—are explored in depth, along with how problems at different levels can produce anxiety and the therapies that can be used to restore balance. Among the featured therapies in this chapter is Family Systems Therapy, an innovative technique to address transgenerational issues that is widely practiced in Europe and just beginning to become known in the United States. This chapter provides a framework for approaching recovery from anxiety as well as for understanding how the natural medicine therapies described in the chapters to follow work to address the whole person.

Chapters 4, 5, and 6 look at three different kinds of energy-based medicine: traditional Chinese medicine, homeopathy, and flower essence therapy. Unlike drugs or nutritional supplements, which operate on a biochemical or physical level, these therapies function on an energetic level to restore the equilibrium of the body, mind, and spirit and dispel anxiety in the process. Energy medicine is little understood in the West, and these chapters present the power of this form of medicine in clear and accessible language.

In chapter 7, we move on to the emotional components of anxiety and the concept of cellular memory—how trauma, both physical and emotional, is stored in the very tissues of the body. The soma (body) therapies covered here—CranioSacral Therapy, SomatoEmotional Release, and Visceral Manipulation—work to release the stored trauma and correct structural misalignment (from birth or injury), both of which can contribute to an anxiety disorder.

Chapter 8 also explores the role of trauma in anxiety and details how two energy-based psychotherapies—Thought Field Therapy and Seemorg Matrix Work—can resolve trauma from the past far more quickly than standard psychotherapeutic methods. These leading-edge therapies, which came onto the psychotherapeutic scene in the 1990s, were both developed by psychotherapists who were frustrated by the lack of results in standard practice. Thought Field Therapy has already gained a reputation for its ability to halt an anxiety attack, while an increasing number of practitioners are seeking training in Seemorg Matrix Work as they learn of its efficiency in clearing psychological trauma.

The last chapter in part 2 focuses on psychospiritual contributions to anxiety and turns to psychic and shamanic healing for the insightful analysis of anxiety and its causes offered by these disciplines. Psychic healing, also known as spiritual healing, considers the role of foreign energies in preventing spiritual connection and stimulating anxiety. Shamanic healing provides an illuminating view of anxiety as disconnection from one's sense of purpose, a condition that is pervasive in the Western world and contributing to our epidemic of anxiety.

The combination of therapies found in these chapters and covering the spectrum of body, mind, and spirit factors in anxiety disorders is unique. By offering a comprehensive and deep approach to healing, these therapies have the potential to help you find your way to a life free of the anxiety and fear that prevent you from living fully.

Natural Medicine Therapies Covered in Part II

Chapter	Health Practitioner	Therapies
3	Dietrich Klinghardt, M.D., Ph.D.	APN (Applied Psycho-neurobiology) Chelation/heavy metal detoxification Family Systems Therapy NAET (allergy elimination) Neural Therapy Thought Field Therapy
	Thomas M. Rau, M.D.	Neural Therapy
4	Ira J. Golchehreh, L.Ac., O.M.D.	Traditional Chinese medicine Acupuncture Herbal medicine
5	Judyth Reichenberg-Ullman, N.D., L.C.S.W.	Constitutional homeopathy
	Carola M. Lage-Roy	Homeopathic nosodes
6	Patricia Kaminski	Flower Essence Therapy
7	Zannah Steiner, C.M.P., R.M.T.	CranioSacral Therapy Visceral Manipulation SomatoEmotional Release
8	Tony Roffers, Ph.D.	Seemorg Matrix Work Thought Field Therapy
9	Rev. Leon S. LeGant	Spiritual/psychic healing
	Malidoma Patrice Somé, Ph.D.	Shamanic healing

The Basics of Anxiety

1 What Is Anxiety and Who Suffers from It?

Every year in the United States, more than 19 million people are suffering from an anxiety disorder. Of these, 6.3 million have a specific phobia such as fear of flying, 5.3 million are afflicted with social anxiety disorder (also known as social phobia), 5.2 million have posttraumatic stress disorder (PTSD), 4 million have generalized anxiety disorder (GAD), 3.3 million have obsessive-compulsive disorder (OCD), and 2.4 million suffer from panic disorder.[11]

While these numbers make anxiety disorders the most common mental illness in the United States today, that unfortunately does not translate into widespread understanding of the disorder. On average, people with anxiety disorders see ten doctors before they finally get a diagnosis,[12] and less than a third of those afflicted receive "appropriate treatment."[13] Since the latter phrase conventionally refers to psychiatric medication with or without attendant psychotherapy, that means that even those who seek help are likely getting, at best, management of their symptoms.

While public awareness of depression as an illness has increased, due in part to the media flurry surrounding Prozac making depression a household word, anxiety is still regarded by many as a psychological failing and a less serious condition than depression. In actuality, the conventional medicine view

Types of Anxiety

The following are the types of anxiety disorders and the number of people in the United States who suffer from them annually:

Specific phobia: 6.3 million

Social anxiety disorder: 5.3 million

Posttraumatic stress disorder (PTSD): 5.2 million

Generalized anxiety disorder (GAD): 4 million

Obsessive-compulsive disorder (OCD): 3.3 million

Panic disorder: 2.4 million

of anxiety disorders is akin to that of depression; that is, they are biologically based brain disorders that have potentially grave consequences for the individual and for society.

An anxiety disorder is far beyond the nervousness or anxiousness we all feel at various times in our lives. While the different types of disorders have their own symptomatology, one prevailing characteristic is shared by all: irrational and excessive fear and dread.[14] This fear and dread can interfere with every aspect of a person's life. At its most severe, it railroads career, social life, and intimate relationships. It can also lead to psychiatric hospitalization. In fact, people with anxiety disorders are six times more likely to undergo such hospitalization than people who do not have anxiety disorders.[15] They are also at greater risk of suicide. Further, anxiety disorders worsen over time if untreated.

Not only are anxiety disorders the most common among mental illnesses, they also carry the highest price tag at $42 billion a year, which is nearly one-third of the total costs for all mental illness.[16] While treatment itself tends to be less expensive than for schizophrenia, for example, the estimated cost in lost productivity from the millions of people suffering from an anxiety disorder comprises about 75 percent of the total costs.[17]

It is clear from these facts that anxiety disorders and the growing epidemic of anxiety in the Western world need to be regarded as a serious problem with serious consequences. At the same time, in the face of these gloomy statistics, it is important to realize that management of symptoms is not the best we can hope for. As you will learn in this book, treating the underlying causes of anxiety poses the opportunity to reverse this epidemic.

The Nature of Anxiety

Anxiety occurs along a spectrum from mild to severe. There is the low-grade anxiety of worry and uneasiness about an event or condition of your life. There is the chronic anxiety of always worrying over something. Then there is the emergency response type of anxiety, which normally occurs in response to a perceived threat. The body's normal reaction to a threat is the fight-or-flight response—the emergency mobilization in which the heartbeat and breathing become rapid, the blood pressure rises, and there is a rush of adrenaline—all of which prepare the individual to act quickly. This response is what happens during an anxiety (panic) attack, but there is no actual threat.

It is clear from these facts that anxiety disorders and the growing epidemic of anxiety in the Western world need to be regarded as a serious problem with serious consequences. At the same time, in the face of these gloomy statistics, it is important to realize that management of symptoms is not the best we can hope for. As you will learn in this book, treating the underlying causes of anxiety poses the opportunity to reverse this epidemic.

Panic attacks may or may not be linked to fearful stimuli, such as taking a plane trip when one suffers from fear of flying. They can strike out of the blue, even during sleep. A panic attack is such a terrifying experience that people can come to "fear the fear," a phenomenon known as anticipatory anxiety. They may begin to curtail their activities to avoid situations that they think might bring on an attack.

A panic attack on its own does not constitute an anxiety disorder, but is part of the symptomatology of such disorders. To meet the official definition of a panic attack, according to the *DSM-IV*, the American Psychiatric Association's diagnostic bible for psychiatric disorders, at least four of the symptoms below must develop quickly and peak within ten minutes in the context of intense fear or discomfort:[18]

• heart palpitations, increased heart rate, or pounding heart

• sweating

• chills or hot flushes

• trembling or shaking

• numbness or tingling

• feeling short of breath or as though one were smothering

• choking feeling

• chest pain or discomfort

• nausea or abdominal distress

• dizziness, lightheadedness, unsteadiness, or faintness

• feeling of unreality or being detached from oneself

• fear of losing control or going crazy

• fear of dying

An anxiety disorder can be likened to allergies in that the response is abnormal in relation to the circumstances. In the case of an allergic reaction, the body mobilizes against a substance that is harmless to most people. In the case of an anxiety disorder, the body mobilizes for no apparent reason or against something that is not objectively threatening.

Types of Anxiety Disorders

In the psychiatric profession, the main diagnostic subcategories of anxiety disorders are panic disorder, specific phobia, social anxiety disorder, generalized anxiety disorder, obsessive-compulsive disorder, and posttraumatic stress disorder. A holistic approach does not use such diagnoses to determine the appropriate treatment course, focusing instead on the particular manifestations and underlying imbalances in the individual patient. Many people receive these labels, however, so it's helpful to know to what they refer.

In regard to the reputed higher prevalence of most of these disorders among women as compared to men, the ratios may not be accurate. Among other factors, women's greater willingness to seek help and the societal onus on men not to admit "weakness" may be skewing the numbers. In addition, men are more apt to mask their anxiety with alcohol and drugs.[19]

> ## In Their Own Words
>
> *"To someone who has not experienced an anxiety disorder, the terror, discomfort, and irrationality associated with this condition will seem incomprehensible. Having lived through it myself, I can say that there are few experiences in life more terrifying or baffling."[22]*
> —Jerilyn Ross, president of the Anxiety Disorders Association of America

Panic Disorder

The *DSM-IV* categorizes panic disorder as two types: with and without agoraphobia. For a diagnosis of either type, the person must have recurrent, unexpected panic attacks, meaning that they seem to come "out of the blue," with at least one month of subsequent worry about having another attack, worry over the consequences, or significant change in behavior connected to the attacks.[20]

Agoraphobia, which translates from the Greek *agora* (marketplace) and *phobos* (fear) as fear of open spaces, is more accurately fear of a place where an attack might occur and from which the person cannot escape, get help, or avoid embarrassment. Typical situations that can raise agoraphobic fears are being away from the home on one's own, in a crowd, standing in a line, on a bridge, or in a car, bus, or train. About a third of the people who have panic disorder suffer from agoraphobia.[21]

A Few Phobias

- acrophobia: fear of heights
- agoraphobia: fear of open spaces
- ailurophobia: fear of cats
- amaxophobia: fear of riding in a car
- apiphobia: fear of bees
- arachnophobia: fear of spiders
- aviophobia: fear of flying
- catagelophobia: fear of being ridiculed
- claustrophobia: fear of confined spaces
- enochlophobia: fear of crowds
- glossophobia: fear of speaking in public
- hemophobia: fear of blood
- hydrophobia: fear of water
- iatrophobia: fear of doctors
- misophobia: fear of dirt or germs
- ophidiophobia: fear of snakes
- ophthalmophobia: fear of being stared at
- pharmacophobia: fear of medicines
- traumatophobia: fear of injury
- trypanophobia: fear of injections
- xenophobia: fear of strangers

Depression, other anxiety disorders, substance abuse, and hypochondriasis (abnormal anxiety about one's health, often with the belief that one has a serious disease, despite lack of medical evidence) are common in panic disorder. Twice as many women as men receive a diagnosis of panic disorder without agoraphobia, and three times as many the agoraphobic type. Onset is usually between late adolescence and the mid-thirties.[23]

Specific Phobia

Formerly known as simple phobia, this form of anxiety is related to identifiable things or situations. Since exposure to the thing or situation generally brings on a panic attack, the person tends to practice avoidance even though they know that the fear is "excessive and unreasonable." The fear may be so great that the person engages in elaborate measures to avoid the phobic stimulus. For a psychiatric diagnosis of this type of anxiety disorder, the person must exhibit distress at having the phobia, and the avoidance, dread, or phobic reaction must significantly interfere with some aspect of the person's life, whether it be career, daily routine, social life, or intimate relationships.[24]

The *DSM-IV* categorizes specific phobias as of the animal type (fear of cats, for example), natural environment type (includes fear of

In Their Own Words

"[I] tried having a couple of drinks before a social situation, thinking that perhaps the alcohol would help. I was very fortunate in that it did not help because if it had, I might have pursued that as a solution."[28]

—CEO of a large corporation who suffered from social anxiety disorder

heights, storms, and water), blood-injection-injury type, situational type (such as fear of flying, taking an elevator, or being in an enclosed place), and other type (includes fear of choking or contracting an illness). People who suffer from a specific phobia often suffer from more than one.[25]

Other anxiety disorders, mood disorders, and substance abuse are common among those with specific phobias. Overall, twice as many women as men are diagnosed with specific phobias. Onset typically occurs in childhood or early adolescence.[26]

Social Anxiety Disorder

Also known as social phobia, this form of anxiety is characterized by fear of social or performance situations involving unfamiliar people or the potential for public scrutiny. Those with social phobia fear being watched and judged by others, behaving in an embarrassing way, or being humiliated by having an evident panic attack. The most commonly reported fear in this disorder is introduction to a stranger.[27] In addition to intense anxiety in this or other problem social situations, the person may blush, break out in a sweat, feel nauseous, tremble, and have trouble talking.

As with the specific phobia, exposure typically brings on an attack, and the person knows that the fear is excessive and unreasonable but practices avoidance anyway. Psychiatric diagnosis requires that the person be distressed at having the phobia or that the avoidance, dread, or phobic reaction significantly interfere with career, daily routine, social life, or intimate relationships.[29]

Other anxiety disorders, mood disorders, substance abuse, and bulimia are conditions that may be paired with social anxiety disorder. The use of alcohol and sedatives such as barbiturates to relieve anxiety is particularly paired with social phobia.[30] The age of onset is generally in midadolescence. Research shows that social anxiety disorder affects both men and women equally, although some study samples reveal that more men than women are afflicted.[31]

Generalized Anxiety Disorder (GAD)

For a diagnosis of GAD, one must suffer from excessive and difficult-to-control anxiety and worry over multiple subjects more days than not for a period of at least six months. In addition, at least three of the following symptoms attend the anxiety and worry, with some present during the entire six-month period cited:[32]

- restlessness, edginess, or a keyed-up feeling

- irritability

- concentration problems or moments of the mind going blank

- easily becoming fatigued

- muscle tension

- sleep problems

Again, distress over one's condition or interference with one's functioning is an additional criterion for diagnosis. It is unusual for a person to suffer from GAD alone; it is most often paired with another anxiety disorder, depression, or substance abuse.[33] Stress-related conditions such as headaches and irritable bowel syndrome are also common among people who suffer from generalized anxiety disorder. The age of onset in more than 50 percent of people with GAD dates from childhood or adolescence; onset after the age of 20 can also occur. Two out of three of those afflicted with GAD are women.[34]

Obsessive-Compulsive Disorder (OCD)

Obsessions are persistent ideas, thoughts, images, or impulses that the person has difficulty ignoring or controlling and which cause distress. Compulsions are repetitive behaviors (such as hand-washing and checking locks) or mental acts (such as counting) aimed at reducing distress or anxiety, often that caused by obsessions. Obsessive-compulsive disorder consists of obsessions or compulsions that take up more than an hour per day, produce obvious distress, or significantly interfere with functioning. As with other anxiety disorders, the person is aware that the obsessions and compulsions are excessive or unreasonable.

> ## In Their Own Words
>
> *"Getting dressed in the morning was tough because I had a routine, and if I didn't follow the routine, I'd get anxious and would have to get dressed again."*[37]
>
> —an OCD sufferer

An example of compulsive behavior is trichotillomania, which is the uncontrollable urge to pull out one's hair. An estimated eight million people in the United States suffer from this disorder.[35]

OCD may coexist with other anxiety disorders, depression, eating disorders, Tourette's disorder, and some personality disorders. OCD occurs equally among adult men and women, but in children, it occurs more frequently in boys than girls. For males, the age of onset is most frequently between 6 and 15 years old, while for females it is between 20 and 29 years old.[36]

Posttraumatic Stress Disorder (PTSD)

Posttraumatic stress disorder involves the reexperiencing of a highly traumatic event, avoidance of associated stimuli, numbing of responsiveness, and increased arousal symptoms such as insomnia, irritability or angry outbursts, hypervigilance, concentration problems, and an exaggerated startle response. Diagnosis requires that the syndrome be present for longer than one month and cause marked distress or significant interference with one's functioning in life.

People who have undergone rape, been in combat, or been the target of incarceration or genocide based on ethnicity or politics have the highest incidence of PTSD among those exposed to traumatic events. Research has found that from one-third to more than 50 percent of these people develop PTSD.[38]

Any age is subject to PTSD. The symptoms may first occur within three months of the trauma or as long as years later. People with PTSD are more likely to suffer from depression, bipolar disorder, substance abuse, and other anxiety disorders (panic disorder, agoraphobia, social phobia, specific phobias, GAD, and OCD).[39]

Anxiety, Comorbidity, and Suicide

Anxiety can be a corollary of other medical conditions (see chapter 2), and there is a comorbidity factor. Comorbidity means that two or more disorders exist together. According to the National Institute of Mental Health (NIMH), about 70 percent of people with an anxiety disorder have another psychiatric problem as well.[40] They are very likely to suffer from depression. For example, more than half of people with panic disorder or OCD also have depression.[41]

One study found that nearly 25 percent of subjects who suffered from seasonal affective disorder (SAD), the "winter blues," also had seasonal panic attacks that disappeared along with the depression with the advent of the longer hours of daylight in the spring.[42] Depression and anxiety coexist so often that the *DSM-IV* included the possibility of a new diagnostic category, called "mixed anxiety-depressive disorder." The overlapping quality of the two disorders is reflected in the fact that many of the underlying causes of anxiety discussed in chapter 2 also produce depression.

 For more about depression, see the author's *The Natural Medicine Guide to Depression* (Hampton Roads, 2003).

As noted throughout the sections on the various types of anxiety disorders, people tend to suffer from more than one kind.

Many people with panic disorder, for example, also have phobias. Substance abuse and eating disorders are common comorbid conditions in anxiety as well.

One study revealed that two-thirds of 102 alcoholic admissions to an alcohol treatment facility suffered from phobic symptoms, with one-third having agoraphobia or a social phobia. Other research demonstrated that in the majority of alcoholic phobics their phobias predated their alcohol dependence.[43]

While many people are aware of the danger of suicide among people with depression, the danger of suicide amongst anxiety sufferers is less widely known. In fact, one study found that the psychiatric patients most apt to commit suicide were those whose ailment was a combination of depression and anxiety.[44]

Research has demonstrated a lifetime rate of suicide attempts of 19.8 percent in people with panic disorders, compared to a rate of 6 percent among those with other mental illnesses, and 0.8 percent in people who don't have a psychiatric disorder. Among people whose panic attacks are below the severity required for a diagnosis of panic disorder, the rate is still high at 12.1 percent.[45] Another study of people with panic disorder found that 42 percent attempted suicide at least once.[46]

The combination of an anxiety disorder with depression or substance abuse puts one at greater risk of suicide. One study found that the incidence of suicide attempts among people with panic disorder was higher if they also suffered from depression and/or substance abuse. Of those with panic disorder combined with major depressive episodes and substance abuse, 72.2 percent attempted suicide; 50 percent of those with panic disorder and either depression or substance abuse did so; 46.2 percent of those with panic disorder and substance abuse; and 17.1 percent of those with panic disorder and neither depression nor substance abuse.[47]

If you or a loved one has an anxiety disorder, it is important to be aware of the warning signs of suicide, so you can act to prevent this tragedy from happening if the signs begin to manifest. A family history of suicide or a previous suicide attempt places one at increased risk of suicide. In addition, the warning signs of suicide are[48]

- feelings of hopelessness, worthlessness, anguish, or desperation

- withdrawal from people and activities

- preoccupation with death or morbid subjects

- sudden mood improvement or increased activity after a period of depression

- increase in risk-taking behaviors

- buying a gun

- putting affairs in order

- thinking, talking, or writing about a plan for committing suicide

If you think that you or someone you know is in danger of attempting suicide, call your doctor or a suicide hotline or get help from another qualified source. Know that there is help and, though it may be difficult to ask for it, a life may depend upon it.

The History of Anxiety

Anxiety disorders have likely plagued humankind throughout time. References to anxiety as a medical condition date back to Greece in the fourth century B.C., with the writings of Hippocrates, the "father of medicine," who prescribed herbs for "nervous unrest."[49] The ancient Greeks also coined the word "agoraphobia" to designate the condition in which otherwise normal people were afraid to leave their houses.[50] In the Bible, we find reference to "abnormal fearfulness."[51]

The names by which anxiety disorders have been known over the centuries include nervous illnesses, nerves, hysteria (in women; hypochondria was considered the equivalent in men), "the vapors," nervous unrest, nervousness, neurasthenia, and anxiety neurosis. Shell shock was an early name for PTSD resulting from war experiences.

In the late 1800s and early 1900s, the German physician Emil Kraepelin studied and documented mental illnesses, providing the foundation for modern psychiatry. Its focus on diagnosis

Famous People Who Had an Anxiety Disorder[56]

Charles Darwin
Sigmund Freud
Abraham Lincoln
John Stuart Mill
Sir Isaac Newton
Nikola Tesla

Actors
Lucille Ball
Olivia Hussey
Sir Laurence Olivier

Writers/Poets/Playwrights
Isaac Asimov
Charlotte Brontë
Robert Burns
Emily Dickinson
John Steinbeck
Alfred, Lord Tennyson
W. B. Yeats

and classification comes from Dr. Kraepelin.[52] The belief that psychological factors were the cause of anxiety arose from the work of Sigmund Freud, however, who in the late 1800s described what he termed "anxiety neurosis." This belief gained cachet in the American medical establishment in the early part of the twentieth century and held sway until the advent of the pharmaceutical age in the latter part of the century.

The various treatments for anxiety conditions through the ages have included herbal medicines, cold-water immersion, hydropathy (heat therapy), bloodletting, the "rest cure," and "nervous clinics." The first manufactured sedative was chloral hydrate, which came into use in 1832.[53] The barbiturate Veronal, introduced in 1904, quickly took hold as the "drug of choice" in private clinics treating nervous conditions.[54] Librium (chlordiazepoxide) was the first antianxiety drug and the first benzodiazepine (a class of tranquilizer) used in psychiatric treatment.[55]

From these pharmaceutical beginnings came a virtual drug explosion, which continues today with the search for new and better anxiolytics (antianxiety drugs) and antidepressants. Psychotherapy was not neglected entirely in this boom. Cognitive therapy, behavioral therapy, and cognitive-behavioral therapy (CBT) were used to good effect with anxiety disorders.

The cognitive approach seeks to change the thinking patterns that contribute to anxiety, while the behavioral approach does the same with patterns of behavior and uses behavioral methods such as exposure therapy to desensitize the individual to the objects or situations that bring on fear. Today, it is widely accepted, due to much research evidence, that these forms of "talk" therapy are particularly beneficial in the treatment of anxiety disorders. They are often used concurrently with medications.

Despite the use of psychiatric drugs and other treatments to address symptoms of anxiety disorder, it wasn't until 1980 that the American Psychiatric Association officially recognized anxiety disorders as a diagnostic category.

The Pharmaceutical Approach to Anxiety

The increasing emphasis on drugs gradually transformed the psychiatric field, shifting the focus of the causality of mental illness from psychological to biochemical and turning the profession into a pharmaceutical industry. While there are quite a few drugs that have long been prescribed for the various anxiety disorders, it wasn't until the 1990s that drugs became the universal panacea for anxiety (and also depression).

In addition to antianxiety drugs, antidepressants are often prescribed for anxiety disorders. In 2000, the Food and Drug Administration (FDA) gave approval for the antidepressant Paxil (paroxetine) to be used specifically in treating social anxiety disorder, the first drug approved for that condition.[57]

In 2001, it approved Paxil for posttraumatic stress disorder. In 2003, the FDA approved the use of Prozac (fluoxetine) for treating children with depression or obsessive-compulsive disorder.[58]

The idea that psychological factors can contribute to anxiety has not been wholly dismissed, but the emphasis in the conventional approach to anxiety, and indeed all psychiatric conditions, is now on medication. There are a number of reasons for this, among which are the pharmaceutical lobby, the shift to a model of biological causality, and the economic strictures of managed care.

The current conventional medical view is that anxiety is a brain disorder caused by an imbalance or dysfunction in neurotransmitters, the brain's chemical messengers that enable communication between cells. Neurotransmitters are the targets of antianxiety drugs (such as Xanax) and antidepressant drugs (such as Prozac), which attempt to manipulate brain chemistry.

Researchers postulate that the problem may center in certain areas of the brain, notably the limbic system. The limbic system of the brain acts as a filter or a kind of switchboard for sensory information and is associated with emotion and behavior. Disturbances in the limbic system can affect mood and, it is thought, contribute to anxiety.

The main components of the limbic system are the amygdala, the hippocampus (a ridge of gray matter, or nerve tissue, in the brain that is involved in memory), and interconnections with the hypothalamus (a supervisory center in the brain that regulates body temperature, blood pressure, metabolism of fats and carbohydrates, blood-sugar level, and emotional expression, among other functions).

> *The current conventional medical view is that anxiety is a brain disorder caused by an imbalance or dysfunction in neurotransmitters, the brain's chemical messengers that enable communication between cells. Neurotransmitters are the targets of antianxiety drugs (such as Xanax) and antidepressant drugs (such as Prozac), which attempt to manipulate brain chemistry.*

The amygdala, an almond-shaped mass of gray matter located deep within the brain, is thought to play a role in arousal, including that of fear. Researchers hypothesize that in anxiety disorders the amygdala is in a hypersensitive state or there is another problem with its circuitry, but this has not been proven and the cause for such dysfunction is unknown.[59] The basal ganglia, a set of four masses of gray matter surrounding the deeper limbic system, which are involved in integrating thoughts, feelings, and movement, may be implicated in anxiety, panic attacks, and especially OCD.[60]

Neither the area of the brain involved nor the role of neurotransmitters in producing anxiety states has been proven, but research suggests that the main neurotransmitters implicated are serotonin, epinephrine/norepinephrine, and GABA (gamma-aminobutyric acid). Part of the "proof" of their involvement comes from the antianxiety effects of making more of these neurotransmitters available in the brain or manipulating their activity, as antianxiety and depressant drugs do. Prozac, for example, acts on serotonin, and Xanax is thought to mimic the action of GABA.

Serotonin is distributed throughout the brain, where it is "the single largest brain system known."[61]

Serotonin, norepinephrine, and dopamine, another neurotransmitter, are monoamines (they are derived from amino acids) and known colloquially as the "feel good" neurotransmitters, meaning that it is their presence and function that allow us to be in a good mood. In addition to influencing mood, serotonin is involved in sensory perception and the regulation of sleep and pain, to name but a few of its numerous activities. Among the symptoms of serotonin deficiency are anxiety, worry, obsessions, compulsions, panic, phobias, insomnia, depression, and suicidal thoughts.[62]

Epinephrine (also known as adrenaline) and norepinephrine (noradrenaline) are hormones produced by the adrenal glands. Norepinephrine is similar to epinephrine and is the form of adrenaline found in the brain.[63] They are involved in the stress response and the physiology of fear and anxiety; an excess has been evidenced in some anxiety disorders.[64]

The amino acid neurotransmitter GABA has a large presence in the brain, being extant in 30 to 50 percent of brain synapses.[65] It operates to stop excess nerve stimulation, thereby exerting a calming effect on the brain. By occupying receptor sites, GABA actually inhibits the transmission of anxiety-related neural messages.[66] Symptoms of deficiency include a stressed and burned-out state, an inability to relax, and tense muscles.[67]

As noted above, neurotransmitters are the targets of psychiatric drugs used in the treatment of mental illness. In the case of anxiety disorders, the drugs typically prescribed are benzodiazepines (tranquilizers), which mimic the action of GABA, and antidepressants, which target the "feel good" neurotransmitters.[68]

The class of drugs known as high-potency benzodiazepines are "new and improved" tranquilizers, such as Valium and Xanax. "When they first came out in the 1960s, benzodiazepines were promoted as relatively safe and free of the well-known addiction problems associated with barbiturates," state psychiatrist Peter R. Breggin, M.D., and David Cohen, Ph.D., authors of *Your Drug May Be Your Problem*. "Nothing could be further from the truth."[69]

In actuality, they are quite addictive and have a range of side effects, which include drowsiness; impairment of coordination, memory, and concentration; and even amnesia.

Tranquilizers work by suppressing brain function. The implications of this are sobering, especially given the dearth of research into the effects of these drugs on the mind over time. "[T]he long-term use of any such drug, especially in high doses, should be viewed as posing a risk of irreversible mental dysfunction,"[70] warn Drs. Breggin and Cohen.

Aside from the dependency issue, the withdrawal reaction from benzodiazepines can involve a return of anxiety symptoms, more severe than they were originally. With a short-acting benzodiazepine such as Xanax, this "rebound effect" can happen daily, say Drs. Breggin and Cohen. "The individual can end up cycling between withdrawal and intoxication from dose to dose throughout the day."[71]

In addition to the negative effects, benzodiazepines do not work to reduce anxiety in one-third of the people who take them.[72] The reason is unknown, so there is no way to tell beforehand if the drug is going to work for you.

Antidepressant drugs are thought to help reduce panic and anxiety as well as depression. For this reason, they are often prescribed for anxiety disorders, even when depression is not an apparent component. There are three classes of antidepressants used in anxiety disorders: SSRIs, tricyclics, and MAOIs.

Prescription Drugs Commonly Used to Control Anxiety Disorders

Anxiolytics (antianxiety drugs)

Benzodiazepines
  Ativan (lorazepam)
  Centrax (prazepam)
  Librium (chlordiazepoxide)
  Klonopin (clonazepam)
  Serax (oxazepam)
  Valium (diazepam)
  Xanax (alprazolam)
Non-Benzodiazepines/azspirone (used for GAD)
  BuSpar (buspirone)

Beta blockers

(to reduce the physiological symptoms of anxiety such as stage fright)
  Inderal (propranolol)
  Tenormin (atenolol)

Antidepressants

SSRIs
  Celexa (citalopram)
  Luvox (fluvoxamine)
  Paxil (paroxetine)
  Prozac (fluoxetine)
  Zoloft (sertraline)

Tricyclics
  Anafranil (clomipramine)
  Aventyl (nortriptyline)
  Elavil (amitriptyline)
  Norpramin (desipramine)
  Pamelor (nortriptyline)
  Pertofrane (desipramine)
  Tofranil (imipramine)

MAOIs
  Nardil (phenelzine)
  Parnate (tranylcypromine)

The SSRIs (selective serotonin re-uptake inhibitors) are typically prescribed for panic disorder, social anxiety disorder, OCD, and PTSD. Prozac and Paxil are in this category. SSRIs block the natural reabsorption of serotonin by brain cells, which boosts the level of available serotonin. SSRIs are relatively new arrivals on the antidepressant scene; Prozac was introduced on the market in 1987.

Earlier categories of antidepressant drugs are tricyclics and monoamine oxidase inhibitors (MAOIs). Tricyclics inhibit serotonin re-uptake, but block norepinephrine re-uptake as well, thus they are less selective than SSRIs. Drugs in this category include clomipramine (Anafranil), which is prescribed for OCD, and imipramine (Tofranil), used for panic disorder and GAD. MAOIs act by inhibiting a certain MAO enzyme that breaks down monoamines; the outcome is more available neurotransmitters.[73] Phenelzine (Nardil) is prescribed for panic disorder and social anxiety disorder. Tranylcypromine (Parnate) is another MAOI that is used for anxiety disorders.[74]

Contrary to popular belief, the newer, more expensive anti-depressants—Prozac, Zoloft, and Paxil—are no more effective than the older antidepressant drugs, according to a report issued by researchers for the U.S. Agency for Health Care Policy and Research and the U.S. Department of Health and Human Services. Not only that, but research has not established that any drug produces better results than psychotherapy, the report reveals.[75]

The reverse is true when it comes to the performance of anti-depressants in cases of anxiety disorder. One NIMH-funded study of 300 people who suffered from panic attacks compared cognitive-behavioral therapy (CBT), antidepressant drugs or placebo pills, and a combination of the two. CBT produced results equal to the drugs over the 12-week trial period, and the combination of drugs and therapy was no better than CBT alone. A six-month follow-up revealed that when the subjects who had received the drugs alone went off the medication at the end of the trial, their symptoms rapidly returned, and by the end of the six months, their condition was no better than those who had been on placebos. The people who had received CBT, however, did not lose the benefits produced by the therapy.[76]

Like benzodiazepines, antidepressants come with a range of side effects, from uncomfortable to untenable, although not everyone who takes the drugs is afflicted. Flattened or dulled feelings and sexual dysfunction are common effects of taking SSRIs. With Prozac, adverse effects include nausea, headaches, insomnia, drowsiness, diarrhea, dry mouth, loss of appetite, sweating, tremors, and rash. Worst of all for anxiety sufferers, Prozac can actually induce anxiety and nervousness.[77]

Research results published in the *International Journal of Psychopharmacology* reported that 15 percent of people taking

Prozac experience this effect.[78] A condition called akathisia (drug-induced agitation) is associated with Prozac-like drugs. In this, panicky agitation, described as like "being tortured from the inside out," prompts pacing, restlessness, and even suicidal urges.[79]

Further, while many people are on antidepressants for years, there has been little research on the long-term effects of taking SSRIs. It is known, however, that they can produce neurological disorders, and permanent brain damage is a danger.[80]

Perhaps the most important argument against the use of antianxiety, antidepressant, and other pharmaceuticals as treatment for anxiety disorders is that they are *not* a treatment. They do nothing to address the deeper causes of anxiety. If the neurotransmitters are indeed out of balance, what caused that to happen? And if that cause is not corrected in treatment, isn't it likely that the neurotransmitters will become imbalanced again after the individual stops taking the drug presumed to compensate for the imbalance? What other factors are involved in this particular person's anxiety disorder? Chapter 2 explores the many causes, triggers, and contributing factors in anxiety, which can serve as a starting point for answering these questions.

2 Causes, Triggers, and Contributors

As with other mental illnesses, the cause of anxiety disorders is unknown. They seem to run in families, but whether this is due to nature (a genetic susceptibility or vulnerability) or nurture (environmental factors) again is unknown. The prevailing medical view that neurotransmitter or brain region dysfunction is behind anxiety has not been proven.

The natural medicine view of anxiety disorders, as of other illnesses, is that imbalances in the body, mind, and/or spirit combine to produce a particular cluster of symptoms in the individual. Inherited vulnerability and environmental factors can be involved in creating these imbalances.

Given that anxiety is epidemic in the world today, it is safe to say that genetics are not the major source of the problem. By definition, genetic disorders affect a stable percentage of the population. A huge jump in the incidence of a disorder signals that other factors are involved. An evolutionary maladaptation to stress cannot account for the epidemic either, because the increase in the number of people suffering from anxiety disorders occurred too rapidly—in a matter of decades.

While successful treatment depends on addressing the underlying factors in each individual, the epidemic suggests that shared environmental factors are operational. Environmental in this usage simply means not genetic, so toxins, psychological trauma, and nutritional deficiencies from a poor diet, for example, all fall in the environmental category. With an inherent vulnerability, one too

20 Causes of Anxiety

The following factors can produce, trigger, or contribute to anxiety:

chemical toxicity

heavy metal toxicity

Candida overgrowth

food allergies

intestinal dysbiosis

sensitivity to food additives

methyl imbalance

nutritional deficiencies and imbalances

neurotransmitter deficiencies or dysfunction

structural factors

hormonal imbalances

medical conditions

medications

street drugs and alcohol

caffeine and nicotine

exercise factors

lack of light

stress

energy imbalances

psychospiritual issues

many environmental stressors can tip the balance of what the system can bear, and an anxiety disorder can ensue.

There is no doubt that modern life exposes us to multiple stressors, from the toxins in our food, air, water, and soil to the hectic pace of the technological age to the fear engendered by our increasingly violent world. While we obviously can't eliminate all of our environmental stressors, we can take steps to reduce our load. While it may not be possible to determine a direct causal link between an individual's anxiety disorder and the environmental factors present in that person's life, when the condition is resolved by identifying and removing or ameliorating those factors, it is safe to say that one or more of them was implicated. It is important to know that the combination of factors differs and the specifics of each factor vary from person to person because no two people have the exact same constitution or emotional and psychological makeup.

The approach of identifying and addressing underlying imbalances has far-reaching benefits for your health in general. Many of the causes discussed in this chapter contribute to a range of disorders in addition to anxiety. Reducing the total burden of stressors in your life is a wise strategy for preventing illness.

This chapter looks at 20 causes or contributing factors in anxiety disorders. While the individual causes may seem to be predominantly physical, psychological, or spiritual in nature, keep in mind that each has reverberating effects on the other levels because body, mind, and spirit are integrally linked.

1. Chemical Toxicity

Toxic overload may be one of the reasons why anxiety has risen so dramatically in the past 40 years. Humans today are exposed to an unprecedented number of chemicals. Testing of anyone on Earth, no matter how remote the area in which they live, will reveal that they are carrying at least 250 chemical contaminants in their body fat.[81]

The onslaught of chemicals begins in the womb, with the transmission of toxins from the toxic mother to the fetus, and continues with breast-feeding. An infant in the United States or Europe imbibes "the maximum recommended lifetime dose of dioxin" in only six months of nursing. Dioxin, a pesticide by-product, is one of the most toxic substances on Earth.[82] The point is that we start life with an already accumulating toxic load.

In their report, *In Harm's Way: Toxic Threats to Child Development,* the Greater Boston Physicians for Social Responsibility summarize research on lead, mercury, cadmium, manganese, nicotine, pesticides (many of which are commonly used in homes and schools), dioxin and PCBs (polychlorinated biphenyls; both PCBs and dioxin stay in the food chain once they enter it, as they pervasively have), and solvents used in paint, glue, and cleaning products.

The report notes that in one year alone (1997), industrial plants released more than a billion pounds of these chemicals directly into the environment (air, water, and land). Further, almost 75 percent of the top 20 chemicals (those released in the largest quantities) are known or suspected to be neurotoxicants.[83] (Neurotoxicants, or neurotoxins, are substances that are toxic to the brain and the nervous system in general.)

Other sources report that of 70,000 different chemicals being used commercially only 10 percent have been tested for their effect on the nervous system.[84]

In addition to the pesticides used directly on crops, the chemicals in the air, water, and soil are fully integrated into our food supply.

Chemical toxicity is known to produce anxiety. The *DSM-IV* cites "toxin exposure" as one of the causes of anxiety disorders.[85]

Chemical toxicity is known to produce anxiety. The *DSM-IV* cites "toxin exposure" as one of the causes of anxiety disorders. According to the National Institute for Occupational Safety and Health, exposure to "harmful substances" accounted for 30 percent of the occupational anxiety, stress, or neurotic disorders leading to time away from work.

According to the National Institute for Occupational Safety and Health, exposure to "harmful substances" accounted for 30 percent of the occupational anxiety, stress, or neurotic disorders leading to time away from work.[86]

Anxiety is a common symptom associated with multiple chemical sensitivity (MCS), a condition of reactivity that is on the severe end of the continuum of the effects of chemicals on the mind and body. One study found that people with MCS have a higher "anxiety sensitivity" than people without MCS. Anxiety sensitivity is a heightened response to feeling anxious, which is typical of anxiety disorders.[87] Other research reveals that approximately half of those with MCS meet the criteria for anxiety disorders and depressive conditions.[88]

The rest of us who are not yet so overtly sensitive are still absorbing the effects of the toxic substances in our environment, and those chemicals are exerting their influence on us. Chemicals to which we are regularly exposed can disturb the production and function of neurotransmitters, block their receptor sites, and prevent enzymes from working.[89]

Consider the hydrazines, a family of widely used chemicals, notably in pesticides, jet fuels, and growth retardants. Hydrazine is sprayed on potatoes to prolong their shelf life. In the body, this chemical blocks serotonin production by blocking the action of vitamin B_6, which is needed at every step in the series of enzyme actions required in the manufacture of serotonin. In just one bag of potato chips or one serving of fast-food French fries, there is sufficient hydrazine to knock out all the B_6 in your body.[90]

2. Heavy Metal Toxicity

The heavy metal mercury has been recognized for centuries as a neurotoxin. Early hatmakers contracted what was known as "mad hatter's disease," the result of poisoning from the mercury used in hatmaking, hence the saying, "mad as a hatter." Anxiety as one of the effects of mercury poisoning is well documented.

Physiologically, mercury's effects on the brain arise from its ability to bond firmly with structures in the nervous system, explains Dietrich Klinghardt, M.D., Ph.D., whose work is featured in chapter 3. Research shows that it is taken up in the peripheral nervous system by all nerve endings (in the tongue, lungs, intestines, and connective tissue, for example) and then transported quickly via nerves to the spinal cord and brainstem.

"Once mercury has traveled up the axon, the nerve cell is impaired in its ability to detoxify itself and in its ability to nurture itself," says Dr. Klinghardt. "The cell becomes toxic and dies—or lives in a state of chronic malnutrition. . . . A multitude of illnesses, usually associated with neurological symptoms, result."[91]

Mercury is bioaccumulative, which means that it doesn't break down in the environment or in the body. The result is that it is everywhere in our environment, in our food, air, and water, and each exposure adds to our internal accumulation. Many of us also carry a source of mercury in our mouths in the form of dental fillings; so-called silver fillings are actually comprised of over 50 percent mercury. These fillings leach mercury, predominantly in the form of vapor, 80 percent of which is absorbed through the lungs into the bloodstream. Chewing raises the level of vapor emission and it remains elevated for at least 90 minutes afterward.[92]

Among the symptoms that improve after having mercury amalgam fillings replaced with nontoxic composite fillings are anxiety, nervousness, irritability, insomnia, depression, fatigue, lack of energy, headaches, memory loss, lack of concentration, allergies, gastrointestinal upset, and thyroid problems.

The heavy metals copper and lead can also cause anxiety.[93] Copper is found in dental fillings, often added as an alloy to gold fillings. Other sources of copper exposure are cigarettes, cookware, and water pipes. Lead exposure is often an occupational hazard; approximately one million Americans are exposed to lead on the job.[94] Other sources of exposure include certain glazed ceramics, old paint, water pipes, fertilizers, and soft vinyl products.

3. Candida Overgrowth

Anxiety, depression, and fatigue are three of the most common effects of an intestinal overgrowth of *Candida albicans,* the yeastlike fungus normally found in the body.[95] The fungus, through its normal metabolic processes, releases substances that are toxic to the brain and interfere with neurotransmitter activity.[96] As noted in the section on Intestinal Dysbiosis to follow, bacteria, yeast, and other substances in the intestines can travel to the brain via the bloodstream. With *Candida* overgrowth, the intestinal lining becomes inflamed, which interferes with the absorption of nutrients.[97] As discussed later, nutritional deficiencies are implicated in anxiety.

Candida overgrowth occurs when something intervenes to disturb the normal balance of flora in the intestinal environment. The main culprit in throwing off the balance is antibiotics, particularly the repeated use of antibiotics, which kill all the beneficial bacteria that keep potentially harmful flora such as *Candida* in check. Weakened immunity may also be a factor in yeast overgrowth.

Eliminating foods that "feed" *Candida* is a common treatment approach to restoring intestinal balance. The so-called Candida diet emphasizes avoiding all forms and sources of sugar, including fruit and fruit juice, carbohydrates, and fermented yeast products.

A number of natural medicine practitioners, notably Thomas Rau, M.D., (see chapter 3) have discovered the connection between *Candida* and mercury, postulating that one of the functions of the fungus in the body is to deal with heavy metals such as mercury, for which it has a particular affinity. If there is a high level of mercury in the body, *Candida* multiplies. Until you detoxify the body of the mercury, says Dr. Rau, you won't be able to get rid of the *Candida* overgrowth on any lasting basis, no matter how perfect your diet or what antifungal drug or natural substance you take. The fungus will just keep coming back.[98]

4. Food Allergies

Food allergies produce a wide range of symptoms and conditions, including anxiety, depression, and other mental disorders. Among the allergenic (allergy-producing) foods linked to panic attacks are wheat, eggs, dairy, chocolate, nuts, melon, strawberries, and bananas.[99] Many people are not aware that they are suffering from food allergies, as the symptoms are often not clearly linked with ingestion of the food, as is the case when someone breaks out in a rash after eating strawberries or experiences a dangerous constriction of their air passages after eating shellfish.

A discussion of allergies involves both what happens in the body on a physical level as well as the imbalance in the energy field that an allergy entails. The latter is why NAET (Nambudripad's Allergy Elimination Techniques; see chapter 3), which employs acupuncture among other techniques to restore the body's energy flow in relation to the allergen (a substance to which one is sensitive or allergic), is effective in eliminating allergies. Disturbances in the flow of energy by themselves produce a range of symptoms, including anxiety, as is detailed in many of the chapters in part 2.

Seeming allergies may actually be intolerances or sensitivities resulting from compromised immune and digestive systems or energy disturbances. Once these factors are eliminated or eased, the food intolerances may disappear.

Food intolerances occur when the body doesn't digest food adequately, which results in large undigested protein molecules entering the intestines from the stomach. When poor digestion is chronic, these large molecules push through the lining of the intestines, creating the condition known as leaky gut, and enter the bloodstream. There, these substances are out of context, not recognized as food molecules, and so are regarded as foreign invaders.

The immune system sends an antibody (also called an immunoglobulin) to bind with the foreign protein (antigen), a process that produces the chemicals of allergic response. The antigen-antibody combination is known as a circulating immune complex, or CIC. Normally, a CIC is destroyed or removed from the body, but under conditions of weakened immunity, CICs tend to accumulate in the blood, putting the body on allergic alert, if you will. Thereafter, whenever the person eats the food in question, an allergic reaction follows.

The intestinal dysfunction inherent in food allergies itself contributes to anxiety, as discussed in the next section.

It is important to consider here the concept of "brain allergies." Until recently, allergies were thought to affect only the mucous membranes, the respiratory tract, and the skin. A growing body of evidence indicates that an allergy can have profound effects on the brain and, as a result, behavior. An allergy or intolerance that affects the brain is known as a brain allergy or a cerebral allergy.

5. Intestinal Dysbiosis

Intestinal dysbiosis means an imbalance of the flora that normally inhabit the intestines. Among these flora are the beneficial bacteria (known as probiotics) *Lactobacillus acidophilus* and *Bifidobacterium bifidum,* potentially harmful bacteria such as *E. coli* and *Clostridium,* and the fungus *Candida albicans,* as discussed previously. Anti-inflammatory drugs, antibiotics, food allergies, and a poor diet can all contribute to disturbing the balance among these flora.

When the balance is disturbed, the microorganisms held in check by the beneficial bacteria proliferate and release toxins that compromise intestinal function. This has far-reaching effects in the body and on the mind. Research has revealed that what passes through the lining of the intestines (see Food Allergies) can make its way through the bloodstream to the brain.[100] As an example of just one of the results of this relationship, in the brain certain intestinal bacteria can interfere with neurotransmitter function,[101] which can contribute to anxiety.

Gastrointestinal complaints such as diarrhea, constipation, gas, and stomach pains are common in anxiety disorders. A survey of more than 13,000 people with panic disorder, for example, revealed that the rate of gastrointestinal symptoms was significantly higher than in the general population.[102]

Anxiety and intestinal conditions are inversely related. For instance, one of the symptoms of irritable bowel syndrome (also characterized by abdominal cramping, diarrhea, and constipation) is anxiety.[103] Conversely, chronic anxiety can produce this condition.[104]

6. Sensitivity to Food Additives

Food additives can produce a range of effects from anxiety, nervousness, hyperactivity, depression, and insomnia to dizziness, blurred vision, and migraines. Research has established that aspartame (an artificial sweetener), aspartic acid (an amino acid in aspartame), glutamic acid (found in flavor enhancers and salt substitutes), and the artificial flavoring MSG (monosodium glutamate) are neurotoxins.[105]

Aspartame and MSG are particularly implicated in anxiety. Panic attacks are well-documented reactions to ingestion.[106]

Aspartame alters amino acid ratios and blocks serotonin production.[107] MSG has been shown to affect serotonin levels.[108]

The more than 3,000 additives used in commercially prepared food have not been tested by their manufacturers for their effects on the nervous system or on behavior.[109] In addition to those mentioned above, common food additives are artificial flavoring, artificial preservatives (BHA, BHT, and TBHQ are in this category), artificial coloring/food dyes, thickeners, moisteners, and artificial sweeteners.

Sensitivity to food additives varies; a high sensitivity may reflect an already large toxic load or weakened immunity. By noticing if your anxiety-related symptoms worsen after ingesting certain foods, you can start the process of elimination for determining which additives, if any, are problematic for you.

7. Methyl Imbalance

Many people who suffer from a combination of anxiety and depression are overmethylated, states biochemical researcher William J. Walsh, Ph.D., chief scientist at the Health Research Institute and Pfeiffer Treatment Center (HRI-PTC) in Warrenville, Illinois.[110] Methyl is one of the more common organic chemicals in the body; methyl groups are present in most enzymes and proteins. Methylation is the process by which methyl groups are added to a compound, making methyl available for the many reactions for which it is needed in the body.

With too much methyl (overmethylation), the body overproduces the three neurotransmitters serotonin, dopamine, and norepinephrine. With too little methyl (undermethylation), the neurotransmitter levels are too low. Folic acid, a member of the B-vitamin family, aids in the manufacture of brain neurotransmitters and needs to be available in the proper ratio with methyl.

In addition to anxiety and depression, chemical and food sensitivities are often present in overmethylation, as are deficiencies in folates (a form of folic acid), vitamin B_3 (niacin), and vitamin B_{12} (cobalamin). Further, someone who is overmethylated is likely to have "an adverse reaction to serotonin-enhancing substances such as Prozac, Paxil, Zoloft, St. John's wort [antidepressant herb], and SAMe [S-adenosyl methionine, antidepressant supplement]," states Dr. Walsh.[111] This fact highlights the need for individualized treatment, rather than automatically using a drug or even a natural remedy applicable to a certain disorder.

Undermethylation is the problem in many people with obsessive-compulsive disorder, says Dr. Walsh. Attendant characteristics include seasonal allergies, deficiencies in calcium, magnesium, and vitamin B_6 (pyridoxine), and an excess of folic acid.

Undermethylation and overmethylation can be detected via blood testing and corrected through a protocol of supplements designed for that purpose and tailored to the individual's particular biochemical status.

Resources Two places that do the blood testing and biochemical treatment for methylation problems are Health Research Institute and Pfeiffer Treatment Center (HRI-PTC), 4575 Weaver Pkwy., Warrenville, IL 60555; tel: 630-505-0300; website: www.hriptc.org; and Olive Garvey Center for Healing Arts, Center for the Improvement of Human Functioning International, 3100 N. Hillside, Wichita, KS 67219; tel: 316-682-3100; website: www.brightspot.org.

8. Nutritional Deficiencies and Imbalances

Nutritional deficiencies and imbalances can affect every body system and produce a range of physical and emotional symptoms, including anxiety. Unfortunately, the psychiatric profession for the most part fails to address this factor in the treatment of mental disorders. The nutrients most implicated in anxiety are amino acids, the B vitamins, and calcium.

No two people with an anxiety disorder will have the exact same nutritional condition. Blood chemistry analysis can determine the precise status of your nutrient levels. With this information, therapeutic intervention can then be tailored to your specific nutrient needs. Random supplementation may not address those needs and may even contribute to further skewing of nutrient ratios.

Amino Acids: The production of neurotransmitters requires the presence of certain amino acids or precursors. For example, tryptophan is the amino acid precursor for serotonin, and GABA is an amino acid that also acts as a neurotransmitter.

Amino acids are the basic building blocks of protein. The body does not manufacture most of the amino acids it requires, so they must be obtained through protein in the diet. With a deficient diet, the body is not able to produce sufficient neurotransmitters, and mental symptoms can be the result.

Amino acid supplementation can be effective in alleviating anxiety and serves as a safe and far less expensive alternative to prescription drugs. Although it may not address the root cause of amino acid deficiency, such as a poor diet, it corrects the problem, unlike drugs. It also increases the supply of neurotransmitters naturally, by simply supplying the body with the building materials it needs, instead of forcing the brain and the neurotransmitters into unnatural function to keep the neurotransmitters available.

Research has found that tryptophan supplementation can be beneficial in the treatment of anxiety, panic disorder, mania, depression, sleep disorders, and psychosis.[112] In the body, tryptophan is converted into 5-HTP (5-hydroxy tryptophan) and then into serotonin. A plant extract form of 5-HTP, available as a supplement, can also be used to boost serotonin levels. Several studies have found that 5-HTP supplementation has benefit for anxiety disorders and can decrease the incidence or severity of panic attacks. In one study, nine of ten subjects with panic attacks, agoraphobia, or GAD experienced significant improvement in their symptoms from taking 5-HTP during the 12-week trial.[113] (Note: high dosages of 5-HTP may produce nausea, other gastrointestinal distress, and drowsiness.)

GABA supplementation has been employed in the treatment of anxiety, nervous tension, stress, acute agitation, hyperactivity, mania, and insomnia, among other disorders.[114]

Vitamins and Minerals: The B vitamins are of particular

importance in the prevention of anxiety, as nervous system health depends upon an adequate supply. In addition, they aid in lowering a high blood level of lactic acid (see Exercise Factors), which has been linked to anxiety and panic attacks.[115]

Specific B-vitamin deficiencies associated with anxiety are vitamin B_1 (thiamin), B_3 (niacin/niacinamide), and B_6 (pyridoxine), all of which are vital to neurotransmitter function. Vitamin B_1, in particular, is known as the "morale vitamin" due to the effects it exerts on mental state and the nervous system.[116] In addition, the *DSM-IV* cites a vitamin B_{12} (cobalamin) deficiency as one of the medical conditions that can produce anxiety symptoms.[117] As B vitamins work together and in ratio, it is important when supplementing to make sure that you get the full vitamin B-complex.

Deficiencies in calcium and magnesium, minerals essential for nerve health, have been linked to anxiety. The mental symptoms of calcium deficiency strongly resemble those of an anxiety attack. In addition, hyperventilation, which tends to occur during a panic attack, actually depletes the blood calcium level. Resulting symptoms include dizziness, confusion, and numbness.[118]

Magnesium is important in itself for nervous system health, and also because it enhances B_6 activity. One of the by-products of magnesium deficiency is a higher level of circulating adrenal hormones, the stress hormones operational during a panic attack. As with calcium, hyperventilation can lead to magnesium depletion.[119]

Research has demonstrated that B-vitamin, calcium, and magnesium supplementation exerts an antianxiety effect.[120] Supplementing with inositol, another member of the B-complex family, has also proven beneficial in reducing anxiety and has been used for that purpose in Europe for years. Early research demonstrated that the brain wave imaging of mental patients taking inositol looked like the brain waves of those on the tranquilizer Librium.[121] Subsequent research showed that inositol decreased both the incidence and severity of pain attacks, and reduced OCD symptoms.[122] Vitamin C supplementation can be useful as well. This may be because the body utilizes large amounts of this important nutrient during stress, so those who suffer from anxiety disorders are likely to be depleted.[123]

Poor diet (such as the standard American diet of processed food) and malabsorption due to gastrointestinal dysfunction are common causes of nutritional deficiencies. The depleted mineral content of the soil in which crops are grown, which translates into food with a lower mineral content than our forebears enjoyed, is a factor as well. Finally, many lifestyle practices and attributes of modern life deplete us of vitamins and minerals, regardless of how well we eat: stress, smoking, alcohol, caffeine, pollution, and heavy metals such as the mercury in our dental fillings.

Given these factors, the recommended daily allowance (RDA; purportedly, the amount of individual vitamins and minerals our body requires daily, whether from food or supplements) is likely far below our nutritive needs, in most cases. The RDA standard is based on a group norm for preventing nutritional deficiencies. There are two problems with that. One, individual needs diverge widely, and two, the level of deficiency the RDAs are designed to avoid is severe. The systems of the body can begin to be compromised long before that degree of deficiency registers. In other words, if you use the RDAs as your guideline, you could be walking around with moderate nutritional deficiencies.

Increasing your intake of foods that contain the nutrients cited above is a good idea if you are prone to anxiety. Note that it is difficult to reverse a deficiency with food alone, however. The following are dietary sources of these nutrients:

- Vitamin B_1: brewer's yeast, wheat germ, sunflower seeds, soybeans, peanuts, liver and other organ meats

- Vitamin B_3: brewer's yeast, rice bran, peanuts, eggs, milk, fish, legumes, avocados, liver and other organ meats

- Vitamin B_6: brewer's yeast, wheat germ, bananas, seeds, nuts, legumes, avocados, leafy green vegetables, potatoes, cauliflower, chicken, whole grains

- Vitamin B_{12}: liver, kidneys, eggs, clams, oysters, fish, dairy

- Calcium: kale, turnip greens, collards, mustard greens, parsley, tofu, kelp, brewer's yeast, blackstrap molasses, cheese, egg yolk, almonds, filberts, sesame seeds, sardines

- Magnesium: parsnips, tofu, buckwheat, beans, leafy green vegetables, wheat germ, blackstrap molasses, kelp, brewer's yeast, nuts, seeds, bananas, avocados, dairy, seafood

- Inositol: citrus, nuts, seeds, legumes

- Vitamin C: green vegetables (particularly broccoli, Brussels sprouts, green peppers, kale, turnip greens, and collards), fruits (particularly guava, persimmons, black currants, strawberries, papaya, and citrus; citrus contains less vitamin C than the other fruits)

9. Neurotransmitter Deficiencies or Dysfunction

The role of neurotransmitters in anxiety is covered in chapter 1. As noted, drug treatment targets these brain chemicals. The focus is on supply rather than function, however. A normal level of a given neurotransmitter does not guarantee that the mind and body will receive its benefits. For example, despite high blood levels of the neurotransmitter serotonin, reduced uptake in the brain may mean that the availability of this vital nerve messenger is actually limited.[124]

As discussed in chapter 1, simply attempting to correct neurotransmitter supply or even function does not address the root problem of why the supply is low or why the neurotransmitters are not working properly. As you will learn in part 2 of this book, treating the root problems, which range from the physical to the spiritual, often results in the neurotransmitter deficiency or dysfunction self-correcting as the body's innate ability to heal itself is restored.

10. Structural Factors

Structural factors such as cranial compression can be a component in anxiety disorders. Such compression, which is the result of skull distortion, can occur through birth trauma or a later physical trauma, such as a car accident. The impact of cranial compression has far-reaching effects throughout the body, but in the head the compression exerts pressure on the brain and cranial nerves, which compromises neurotransmitter function and brain function in general. This factor is explored in depth in chapter 7.

11. Hormonal Imbalances

Hormones "are probably second only to the chemicals of the brain in shaping how we feel and behave."[125] Hormonal imbalances influence brain chemistry and the nervous system. The hormones most often implicated in anxiety are thyroid hormones, pituitary and adrenal hormones, and reproductive hormones. In addition to organic dysfunction, toxic exposure, stress, diet, and exercise can all affect hormonal levels and balance.

Both hypothyroidism and hyperthyroidism (an underactive and overactive thyroid gland, respectively) can underlie anxiety. Hypothyroidism is often overlooked as a cause because it can be at a subclinical level and still produce anxiety.

Both hypothyroidism and hyperthyroidism (an underactive and overactive thyroid gland, respectively) can underlie anxiety. Hypothyroidism is often overlooked as a cause because it can be at a subclinical level and still produce anxiety.

As noted in the previous chapter, an excess of the adrenal stress hormones epinephrine (adrenaline) and norepinephrine (noradrenaline) may be operational in anxiety disorders. Implicated pituitary gland hormones are vasopressin and ACTH (adrenocorticotrophic hormone). When the stress response becomes chronic, the pituitary releases these hormones. Vasopressin constricts blood vessels, causing blood pressure to rise. Research has found that people who suffer from OCD often have higher than normal levels of vasopressin.[126]

ACTH stimulates the adrenal glands to release the stress hormone cortisol, high levels of which have been linked to anxiety disorders.[127]

In women, too little of the hormone estrogen in relation to progesterone tends to produce depression, while too much estrogen in relation to progesterone (a condition known as estrogen dominance) tends to result in anxiety.[128] Estrogen dominance has become more common among women as a result of so-called environmental estrogens (xenoestrogens), which are ubiquitous chemical toxins that, once in the body, mimic the effects of estrogen.

Various studies have demonstrated a link between premenstrual syndrome (PMS) and anxiety, with a range of 30 to 95 percent of healthy women experiencing a premenstrual rise in anxiety.[129] Panic is also a symptom of PMS. As a result, some women receive an anxiety disorder diagnosis when their problem is hormonal. For women with an anxiety disorder with other causes, the time before menstruation can produce an exacerbation of their condition. Again, estrogen dominance is a typical cause of anxiety associated with PMS.[130] Natural progesterone, in an oral or cream form, can help restore the ratio of progesterone to estrogen and reduce anxiety and panic.

12. Medical Conditions

There are a number of medical conditions that can produce the symptoms of anxiety disorders. Among them are hypothyroidism or hyperthyroidism (see Hormonal Imbalances), hyperadrenocorticism (elevated hormonal secretion from the cortex of the adrenal glands), cardiovascular conditions, chronic obstructive pulmonary disease, pneumonia, encephalitis, vitamin B_{12} deficiency, and hypoglycemia (low blood sugar). The symptoms of severe hypoglycemia and those of panic attacks are so similar that misdiagnosis is frequent.[131]

While mitral valve prolapse (MVP), an abnormality in a valve in the heart, has been thought to play a role in anxiety disorders, research suggests that this is not the case. The rate of MVP among people with such disorders is on a par with the rate in the general population.[132] It may be that the heart-related sensations that accompany MVP are more likely to raise anxiety in those who suffer from anxiety disorders than those who do not.

13. Medications

A wide range of prescription medications can cause a substance-induced anxiety disorder. Among them are some of the very drugs taken to alleviate anxiety, notably antidepressants, as discussed in chapter 1. Others are anesthetics, pain relievers, corticosteroids, nonsteroidal anti-inflammatories, antihistamines, bronchodilators, ephedrine, pseudoephedrine, antihypertensives, anticonvulsants, antiparkinsonian medications, antipsychotics, synthetic thyroid hormones, and birth control pills. In addition, withdrawal from antianxiety drugs and sedatives can produce anxiety.[133]

14. Street Drugs and Alcohol

Cocaine, amphetamines, PCP (angel dust), hallucinogens, and inhalants are sources of substance-induced anxiety disorders and can worsen existing symptoms.[134] They affect the biochemistry of the brain. Habitual use of cocaine and amphetamines, for example, can interfere with production of the neurotransmitters that inhibit irritability and other heightened reactivity, leading to excessive anxiety.[135] Narcotics, which people may use in an attempt to self-medicate, to numb symptoms, can actually worsen the anxiety.[136] People with panic disorder frequently cite the use of marijuana as the "single initiatory factor" in the first attack they experienced.[137]

Alcohol interferes with normal neurotransmitter function by impeding the supply of tryptophan to the brain and thus reducing serotonin formation, which, as discussed previously, has implications for anxiety. Habitual drinking of alcoholic beverages is associated with hypoglycemia and nutritional deficiencies, notably B vitamins, vitamin C, folic acid, zinc, potassium, and magnesium.[138] Note the overlap with nutritional deficiencies often present in anxiety disorders.

15. *Caffeine and Nicotine*

In the general population, people who drink a lot of coffee test higher for anxiety and depression and are also more likely than their more abstemious counterparts to develop psychotic disorders.[139] Among psychiatric patients, research has found that the level of caffeine ingested is positively correlated with the degree of mental illness,[140] meaning that the more caffeine taken in, the worse the symptoms.

Caffeine does a lot more than give you a jittery edge. It actually affects your neurotransmitters, stimulating the release of norepinephrine and others. As with alcohol, habitual excess intake can leave you with a neurotransmitter deficit, along with hypoglycemia and nutritional deficiencies, as caffeine interferes with the absorption of important nutrients such as B vitamins, magnesium, calcium, potassium, and zinc.[141] Again, a number of these deficiencies are frequently present in anxiety disorders.

Avoiding caffeine or at least limiting intake is thus advisable. Be sure to consider all caffeine sources. Some people give up or cut down on coffee and black tea, but overlook the high caffeine content in colas.

In addition to the known health hazards posed by smoking, nicotine, like stimulants and alcohol, affects neurotransmitters. In the brain, it behaves like acetylcholine, excess levels of which have been linked to anxiety, irritability, muscle twitching, and seizures.[142]

16. *Exercise Factors*

Exercise stimulates the release of mood-regulating neurotransmitters, along with endorphins, chemicals that lift mood and reduce stress level. It increases oxygen, glucose, and nutrient supply to the brain, which improves cerebral function and the ability to cope with stress.[143] Exercise also helps flush toxins out of the body, the benefits of which have been discussed previously.

Exercise can alleviate anxiety, irritability, hyperactivity, insomnia, and depression.[144] As with proper nutrition and sleep, it is a basic need of the body. Lack of exercise is an environmental stressor that is relatively easy to remedy.

In addition to lack of exercise, there is another exercise issue of relevance in anxiety disorders. It involves lactic acid, high blood levels of which have been linked to anxiety.[145] Lactic acid is a substance that forms in the body as a result of muscular activity. Normally, lactic acid is oxidized during exercise due to the increased oxygenation of the blood. One reason that lactic acid accumulates in the body is inadequate oxygenation.

For some people with anxiety disorders, vigorous exercise exacerbates their symptoms. Research has shown that the blood lactate (salt of lactic acid) levels in those who experience this are higher than normal after exercise. In addition, giving lactate to people with panic disorder can bring on a panic attack, whereas it does not do so in people without the disorder.[146] While the reasons for this are not fully understood, it serves as a caution to those with anxiety disorders. Strenuous aerobic exercise may worsen your symptoms. You might consider trying calmer exercise such as walking, yoga, or tai chi.

17. Lack of Light

In this technological age many of us spend the vast majority of our time indoors under artificial light. As a consequence, many of us are not getting enough of the full-spectrum light that characterizes sunlight. Lack of light is linked to anxiety, irritability, decreased ability to cope with stress, emotional instability, hyperactivity, depression, fatigue, and malabsorption of nutrients, among other symptoms and conditions.[147]

Lack of light results in lower levels of serotonin and can contribute to sleep disorders such as insomnia because it interferes with melatonin function. Melatonin, a hormone important in sleep regulation, is manufactured from serotonin.

Spending more time outdoors and using full spectrum light bulbs in your indoor environments are steps you can take to ameliorate this factor.

18. Stress

Anxiety disorders are by nature highly stressful to those who suffer from them. Feeling fear, ranging from the mild to terror, is a stressful experience. Chronic stress wreaks havoc on the body, mind, and spirit and creates a vicious circle. In particular, stress drains nutrients, and the resulting deficiencies compromise the neurochemistry in the brain. This in itself is a factor in anxiety, but it further contributes by reducing the body's ability to handle stress. Stress can also throw off the balance of the energy system of the body, which, again, has the dual contribution to anxiety.

The fact that stress is such a fundamental component of anxiety is a strong argument for reducing the amount of stress in your life wherever possible, whether through avoidance of known stressful situations, making changes in your circumstances or lifestyle, and/or practicing meditation and relaxation techniques. In addition, attending to the other factors in this chapter can significantly reduce your stress load.

19. Energy Imbalances

There are a number of different ways to discuss the flow of energy in the human body. Physiologically, the salient point for anxiety disorders is that the nervous system operates on electrical charges. Extending outward, you could speak of the body's electromagnetic field and the far-reaching effects on mental and physical health caused by disturbances in that field (see chapter 3).

If you regard energy from the perspective of homeopathy, which is an energy-based medicine, illness is regarded as a disturbance in the individual's vital force. Homeopathic remedies restore that vital force to its natural equilibrium, which restores balance to the body, mind, and spirit (see chapter 5). If you consider energy from a shamanic or psychic viewpoint, you might explore the presence of foreign energy in an individual's energy field (see chapter 9).

Whatever language you choose to employ to describe the phenomenon, a disturbance in an individual's energy field can contribute to anxiety. The relationship of energy to other factors can be cyclical, with physical factors (such as nutritional deficiencies) or psychological or spiritual issues causing or being caused by a disturbance in energy flow. Part II explains and explores in depth energy imbalances as a factor in anxiety.

20. Psychospiritual Issues

In an article published in the *Psychiatric Times Journal* in December 1996, psychiatrist David Kaiser, M.D., criticized the current solely biological approach to mental illness. "What is left completely out," he wrote, "are any notions that our psychic ills are a reflection of cultural pathology. In fact, this new biologic psychiatry can only exist to the extent it can deny not only the truths of psychoanalysis, but also the truth of any serious cultural criticism. It is then no surprise that this psychiatry thrives in this country presently, where such denials are rampant and deeply embedded."[148]

To ignore the psychological, emotional, and spiritual factors in any illness is to treat only part of a person. As noted in the previous section, psychological, emotional, and spiritual issues have the capacity to throw the energy system out of balance, which can have repercussions on all levels, including the electrical transmission of the nervous system. Thus, treatment that does not address all areas will not produce lasting health.

Psychotherapy is one avenue for exploring the psychological and spiritual dimensions of anxiety. It could be considered psychological and spiritual housecleaning or the maintenance work that taking good care of something requires. Taking good care of yourself means attending to the needs of body, mind, and spirit.

The contribution of the mind and spirit in anxiety is fully explored in part 2. For example, chapter 7 examines how early trauma can be stored in the body as cellular memories that keep anxiety encrypted in the body. Chapter 8 covers the effects of emotional and psychological trauma on energy and the spirit, while chapter 9 looks at the role of spiritual and psychic factors in anxiety.

The next chapter provides a model that will help you make sense of the various levels of healing and how they relate to each other.

Action Plan

As a summary of the information in this chapter, the following are steps you can take to eliminate the causes, triggers, and contributors to your anxiety.

- Reduce your toxic exposure wherever possible. Avoid using toxic house and garden products; eat organically grown food; and drink pure water instead of tap water.

- Reduce your heavy metal exposure by avoiding sources of copper, lead, and mercury wherever possible. You may want to investigate having your mercury dental fillings replaced with nonmercury amalgams; hair analysis and other tests can determine if the level of mercury in your body is high.

- Avoid foods and other substances to which you are allergic, or get allergy treatment such as NAET to eliminate the problem (see chapter 3). If you suspect you have allergies, but don't know to what, NAET can help you identify allergens.

- Address any intestinal or digestive dysfunction, such as an overgrowth of *Candida*. Taking probiotics helps improve digestion.

- Avoid food additives, particularly if your symptoms seem to worsen after ingesting additives.

- Eat a healthful, balanced diet. Avoid junk food, fast food, and processed food.

- Have your biochemical status checked to identify any nutritional deficiencies or imbalances, and take the appropriate supplements to correct them. Consult with a qualifed practitioner of natural medicine to determine if amino acid supplements are indicated.

- Consider consulting a CranioSacral therapist to eliminate structural factors that may be contributing to your anxiety disorder (see chapter 7).

- Have your doctor check you for hormonal imbalances.

- Work with your doctor to determine if you have any medical conditions that produce symptoms of anxiety.

- Consult your doctor about whether any medications you are taking might be contributing to your anxiety disorder. Also ask about any antidepressants you are taking or considering taking; some can exacerbate anxiety.

- Avoid or limit intake of alcohol and caffeine. If you smoke, consider quitting. Avoid recreational drugs, especially stimulants such as cocaine and amphetamines.

- Get regular exercise of a type that doesn't increase your anxiety symptoms.

- Make sure to spend time outdoors every day. If lack of light is a problem for you, consider using full-spectrum light bulbs in your house.

- Find ways to reduce or manage the stress in your life. Meditation and relaxation techniques can be beneficial.

- Address energy imbalances through acupuncture, homeopathy, or other forms of energy-based medicine (see part 2).

- Explore psychospiritual issues through psychotherapy or other modalities (see chapters 3 and 6–10).

PART II

Natural Medicine Treatments for Anxiety

3 A Model for Healing

While many people speak generally of the body-mind-spirit connection, Dietrich Klinghardt, M.D., Ph.D., based in Bellevue, Washington, has developed a detailed paradigm that explains that connection in terms of Five Levels of Healing: the Physical Level, the Electromagnetic Level, the Mental Level, the Intuitive Level, and the Spiritual Level.

Dr. Klinghardt is internationally acclaimed for this brilliant and comprehensive model of healing, for his expertise in Neural Therapy, and for several effective therapeutic techniques he has developed (see "About the Therapies and Techniques" at the end of this chapter). He trains doctors around the world in his model and techniques and is perhaps the person most responsible for bringing Neural Therapy to the attention of the medical and lay communities.

The Five Levels of Healing model provides a comprehensive way to approach and understand many chronic disorders, including anxiety. Health and illness are a reflection of the state of these five levels. Anxiety, like any health problem, can originate on any of the five levels. A basic principle of Dr. Klinghardt's paradigm is that an interference or imbalance on one level, if untreated, spreads upward or downward to the other levels. Thus anxiety can involve multiple levels, sometimes even all five, if the originating imbalance is not correctly addressed.

Another basic principle is that healing interventions can be implemented at any of the levels. Unless upper-level imbalances are addressed, restoring balance at the lower levels will not produce long-lasting effects. This provides an answer to why rebalancing the biochemistry of the brain, correcting nutritional deficiencies, or restoring hormonal health does not resolve some cases of anxiety disorder. Treating these factors only addresses the Physical Level of illness and healing and leaves the causes at the Intuitive Level, for example, intact. The corrected factors will soon be thrown off again by the downward cascade of this imbalance.

The Five Levels of Healing model also provides a useful framework for the natural medicine therapies covered in the rest of this book. You will see that they approach anxiety by identifying and treating disturbances at the different levels. In keeping with the holism of natural medicine, a number of the therapeutic modalities function on several levels. For example, Traditional Chinese medicine (chapter 4) works on both the Physical and the Electromagnetic Levels, while Matrix therapy (chapter 8) works on the Electromagnetic and Mental Levels.

The following sections explore the Five Levels of Healing in detail and identify therapies that can remove various interferences at each level.

The First Level: The Physical Body

The Physical Body includes all the functions on the physical plane, such as the structure and biochemistry of the body. Interference or imbalance at this level can result from an injury or anything that alters the structure, such as accidents, concussions, dental work, or surgery. "Surgery modulates the structure by creating adhesions in the bones and ligaments, which changes the way things act on the Physical Level," says Dr. Klinghardt.

Imbalance at the first level can also result from anything that alters the biochemistry such as poor diet, too much or too little of a nutrient in the diet or in nutritional supplements, or taking the wrong supplements for one's particular biochemistry. Organisms such as bacteria, viruses, and parasites can also change the host's biochemistry. "They all take over the host to some degree and change the host's behavior by modulating its biochemistry," Dr. Klinghardt explains.

"The whole world of toxicity also belongs in the biochemistry," he says. Toxic elements that can alter biochemistry include heavy metals such as mercury, insecticides, pesticides, and other environmental chemicals. Interestingly, heavy metals operate on both the Physical Level and the next level of healing, the Electromagnetic Level. Due to their metallic nature, they can alter the biochemistry by creating electromagnetic disturbances.

All of these factors at the Physical Level—surgery, injury, dental work, nutritional imbalances, microorganisms, heavy metals, and other toxins— can play a role in producing symptoms of mental illness, including anxiety, according to Dr. Klinghardt.

All of these factors at the Physical Level—surgery, injury, dental work, nutritional imbalances, microorganisms, heavy metals, and other toxins—can play a role in producing symptoms of mental illness, including anxiety, according to Dr. Klinghardt.

The therapeutic modalities that function at this level are those that address biochemical or structural aspects, from drug and hormone therapies to herbal medicine and nutritional supplements, as well as mechanical therapies such as chiropractic.

The Second Level: The Electromagnetic Body

The Electromagnetic Body is the body's energetic field. Dr. Klinghardt explains it in terms of the traffic of information in the nervous system. "Eighty percent of the messages go up to the brain [from the body], and 20 percent of the messages go down from the brain [to the body]. The nerve currents moving up and down generate a magnetic field that goes out into space, creating an electromagnetic field around the body that interacts with other fields." Acupuncture meridians (energy channels) and the chakra system are part of the Electromagnetic Body.

A chakra, which means "wheel" in Sanskrit, is an energy vortex or center in the nonphysical counterpart (energy field) of the body. There are seven major chakras positioned roughly from the base of the spine, with points along the spine, to the crown of the head. As with acupuncture meridians, when chakras are blocked, the free flow of energy in the body's field is impeded.

See Also For more about chakras, see chapter 8.

Biophysical stress is a source of disturbance at this level. Biophysical stress is electromagnetic interference from devices that have their own electromagnetic fields, such as electric wall outlets, televisions, microwaves, cell phones, cell phone towers, power lines, and radio stations. These interfere with the electromagnetic system in and around the body.

For example, if you sleep with your head near an electric outlet in the wall, the electromagnetic field from that outlet interferes with your own. An outlet may not even have to be involved. Simply sleeping with your head near a wall in which electric cables run can be sufficient to throw your field off. The brain's blood vessels typically contract in response to the man-made electromagnetic field, leading to decreased blood flow in the brain, says Dr. Klinghardt.

Geopathic stress, or electromagnetic emissions from the earth, is another source of disturbance. Underground streams and fault lines are a source of these emissions. Again, proximity of your bed to one of these sources—for example, directly over a fault line—can throw your own electromagnetic field out of balance and produce a wide range of symptoms. Simply shifting the position of your bed in the room may remove the problem.

Interference at the second level can cascade down to the Physical Level. The constriction of the blood vessels in the brain in response to biophysical or geopathic stress results in the blood carrying less oxygen and nutrients to the brain. The ensuing deficiencies are a biochemical disturbance, with obvious implications for brain function and mental health. If such deficiencies have their root at the Electromagnetic Level, however, it is important to know that you cannot fix them by taking certain supplements to correct the biochemistry, cautions Dr. Klinghardt.

For example, if an individual has a zinc deficiency, supplementing with zinc may correct the problem if it is merely a biochemical disturbance (a first-level issue). If the restriction of blood flow in the brain as a result of sleeping too close to an electrical outlet (a second-level issue) is behind the deficiency, taking zinc may seem to resolve the problem, but it will return when the person stops taking the supplement. Moving the bed away from the outlet will stop the electromagnetic interference and prevent the recurrence of a zinc deficiency.

Physical trauma or scars can also throw off the second level. "If a scar crosses an acupuncture meridian, it completely alters the energy flow in the system," observes Dr. Klinghardt. An infected tooth or a root canal can accomplish the same. Heavy metal toxicity, from mercury dental fillings and/or environmental metals in the air, water, and food supply, can block the entire electromagnetic system. "We know that the ganglia can be disturbed by a number of things, but toxicity in general is often responsible for throwing off the electromagnetic impulses." Vaccinations can have the same effect. (Ganglia are nerve bundles that are like relay stations for nerve impulses.)

The therapies that address this level of healing are those that correct the distortions of the body's electromagnetic field. Acupuncture and Neural Therapy (see "About the Therapies and Techniques" at the end of this chapter) are two strong modalities for this level. Neural Therapy's injection of local anesthetic in the ganglion breaks up electromagnetic disturbances. You could call the local anesthetic "liquid electricity," says Dr. Klinghardt.

Another therapeutic modality that functions at the second level is ayurvedic medicine (the traditional medicine of India). As it employs a combination of herbs and energetic interventions, it actually covers the first two levels of healing: the herbs work on the Physical Level, and the energetic aspect on the Electromagnetic Level.

 For more about acupuncture/traditional Chinese medicine, see chapter 4.

Neural Therapy and Anxiety

Teresa, 45, had suffered from anxiety since she was a teenager. She came from a family of wealthy entrepreneurs and felt great anxiety over what she perceived as her inadequacies. Her whole life was colored by anxiety; it painted her life in gray tones. She would wake up at night and, unable to quiet her mind, lie there with anxiety-laden thoughts going round and round in her head: "I couldn't fulfill expectations in the past, and I won't be able to in the future. I'll never find another husband. No one likes me; what am I doing wrong? Why do I suffer all the time?"

Her marriage had ended in divorce, and her anxiety interfered with her relationships with other people and with her ability to work. Illness was also her constant companion. For 15 years, she had recurrent kidney infections, back pain, and gynecological problems, which ultimately led to a hysterectomy. (It is interesting to note that, according to traditional Chinese medicine, the organ associated with fear is the kidneys.) Between her illnesses and her anxiety, she was frequently unable to function.

It was not anxiety, but yet another severe kidney infection that initially brought Teresa to Thomas M. Rau, M.D., a pioneer of European biological medicine and director for the past ten years of the Paracelsus Klinik in Lustmühle, Switzerland. European biological medicine draws from a wide range of therapeutic modalities to restore the chemistry and internal balance of the body, including acupuncture/traditional Chinese medicine, Neural Therapy, and homeopathy, among numerous others.

In talking with Teresa, Dr. Rau learned that anxiety had been a lifelong problem for her. The combination of this, the recurrent kidney problems, her low self-esteem, and a tendency to dwell on the past indicated deficient energy on the Kidney meridian, according to Chinese medicine. As this meridian transports *jing,* or life essence, a compromise of its energy flow has a strong impact on one's attitude toward life.

Dr. Rau's treatment focused on upbuilding the Kidney meridian, getting the energy to flow more strongly. To accomplish this he used Neural Therapy, injecting homeopathic preparations into a meridian point located in the lower abdomen and into the kidneys themselves via injections in the back over the kidney area. The homeopathic preparations were of two plants: horsetail (*Equisetum arvense*) and goldenrod (*Solidago virgaurea*).

Horsetail has a long tradition of use in herbal medicine for urinary disease, while goldenrod is indicated for urinary infections in which nervousness and restlessness are present.[149] Homeopathic goldenrod is indicated for chronic kidney conditions. In reference to its ability to restore *jing,* Dr. Rau calls goldenrod "the plant of life." It counteracts the gray "Why me?" attitude and fortifies the "I am as I am" attitude. This speaks to the classic complaint of this type of kidney patient: "Nobody likes me. What's wrong with me?" Homeopathic horsetail works to fortify confidence and self-esteem.

Teresa had about 20 Neural Therapy injections over two years. Her condition required this many treatments because of its chronic, severe, and long-standing nature. Gradually, as the Kidney meridian's energy flow was restored, Teresa's anxiety subsided, as did her kidney problems. Her self-esteem increased, too. Dr. Rau notes that energy disturbances can affect the personality. Restoring the flow can actually change the personality profile. In Teresa's case, simply fortifying the Kidney energy "clearly changed her attitude and her life," says Dr. Rau.

No longer crippled by anxiety and physical problems, Teresa began to function well in the interpersonal and professional arenas, and went on to head one of the family businesses. It has now been seven years since she completed treatment, and she has not had a kidney infection nor an anxiety attack in that time.

 For information about and referral to practitioners of biological medicine, contact the Biological Medicine Network, c/o Marion Foundation, 3 Barnabas Rd., Marion, MA 02738; tel: 508-748-0816; e-mail: bmn@marionfoundation.org.

The Third Level: The Mental Body

The third level is the Mental Level or the Mental Body, also known as the Thought Field. This is where your attitudes, beliefs, and early childhood experiences are. "This is the home of psychology," says Dr. Klinghardt. He explains that the Mental Body is outside the Physical Body, rather than housed in the brain. "Memory, thinking, and the mind are all phenomena outside the Physical Body; they are not happening in the brain. The Mental Body is an energetic field."

Disturbances at this level come from traumatic experiences, which can begin as early as conception. Early trauma or an unresolved conflict situation leaves faulty circuitry in the Mental Body, explains Dr. Klinghardt. For example, if at two years old, your parents divorced and your father was not allowed by law to see you, you may have formed the beliefs that your father didn't love you and that it was your fault your parents broke up because you are inherently bad. These damaging beliefs are faulty mental circuitry.

The mind replays traumatic experiences over and over, keeping constant stress signals running through the autonomic nervous system. These disturbances trickle down and affect the Electromagnetic Level of healing, changing nerve function by triggering the constriction of blood vessels, and in turn, affecting the biochemical level in the form of nutritional deficiency.

It may look like a biochemical disturbance, says Dr. Klinghardt, but the cause is much higher up. "Again, this is a situation you cannot treat with lasting results by giving someone supplements, Neural Therapy, or acupuncture." You have to address the third-level interference, the problem in the Mental Body.

Despite what people may conclude from the related names, so-called mental disorders aren't necessarily a function of disturbance in the Mental Body. The cause can be on any of the five levels, iterates Dr. Klinghardt. In fact, in most cases, the third level is not the source. In his experience, most "mental" disorders arise from disturbances on the fourth level. In all cases, the source level must be addressed or a long-term resolution will not be achieved.

Dr. Klinghardt uses Applied Psychoneurobiology, which he developed, and Thought Field Therapy to effect healing at the third level (see "About the Therapies and Techniques"). Among the other therapeutic modalities that work at this level are psychotherapy, hypnotherapy, and homeopathy.

The Fourth Level: The Intuitive Body

The fourth level is the Intuitive Body. Some people call it the Dream Body. Experience on this level includes dream states, trance states, and ecstasy, as well as states with a negative association such as nightmares, possession, and curses. The Intuitive Body is what the Swiss depth psychologist C. G. Jung called the collective unconscious. "On the fourth level, humans are deeply connected with each other and also with flora, fauna, and the global environment," says Dr. Klinghardt.

The fourth level is the realm of shamanism. Other healers who can work at this level to remove interference are those who practice transpersonal psychology. Stated simply, transpersonal refers to an acknowledgment of the phenomena of the fourth level, "the dimension where a person is affected deeply in themselves by something that isn't of themselves, that is of somebody else. Transpersonal psychology is really a cover-up term for modern shamanism," observes Dr. Klinghardt, meaning that psychotherapists who acknowledge the importance of spiritual connection are facilitating the kind of healing that was traditionally the purview of shamans.

For healing of the Intuitive Body, Dr. Klinghardt uses what is known as Systemic Family Therapy, or Family Systems Therapy. It addresses interference that comes from a previous generation in the family. In this type of interference, he says, "the cause and effect are separated by several generations. It goes over time and space." Rather than a genetic inheritance of a physical weakness, it is an energetic legacy of an injustice with which the family never dealt.

The range of specific issues that can be the source is vast, but it usually involves a family member who was excluded in a previous generation. When the other family members don't go through the deep process of grieving the excluded one, whether the exclusion results from separation, death, alienation, or ostracism, the psychic interference of that exclusion is passed on. Another common systemic factor involves identification with victims of a forebear.

"A member of the family two, three, or four generations later will atone for an injustice," without even knowing who the person involved was or what they did, explains Dr. Klinghardt. For example, a woman murders her husband and is never found out. She marries again and lives a long life. Three generations later, one of her great-grandchildren is born. To atone for the murder, the child self-sacrifices by, for example, developing brain cancer at an early age, being abused or murdered, or starting to take drugs as a teenager and committing a slow suicide.

"It's a form of self-punishment that anybody can see on the outside, but nobody understands what is wrong with this child— he had loving parents, good nutrition, went to a good school, and look what he's doing now, he's on drugs. But if you look back two or three generations, you'll see exactly why this child is self-sacrificing." Dr. Klinghardt notes that mental illness is "very often an outcome on the systemic level."

Systemic Family Therapy involves tracing the origins of current illness back to a previous generation. For the discovery process, Dr. Klinghardt uses the Systemic Family Therapy developed by German psychoanalyst Bert Hellinger. Sometimes an event is known in a family; sometimes it is not. By questioning a client, Dr. Klinghardt is usually able to discover an event from a previous generation that is a likely source of interference for the client's current condition. If no one knew about a certain event, such as the murder in the example above, there are usually clues in a family that point to those people as a possible source.

For the therapy, the client or a close relative chooses audience members to represent the people in question. In our example, they would be the great-grandmother, great-grandfather, and the new husband. These people come together on a stage or central area. They are not told the story, even when the story is known. "They just go up there not knowing anything, and suddenly feel all these feelings and have all these thoughts come up. . . . Very quickly, within a minute or two, they start feeling like the real people in life have felt, or are feeling in their death now, and start interacting with each other in bizarre ways," says Dr. Klinghardt.

The client typically does not participate, but simply observes. "The therapist does careful therapeutic interventions, but there's very little needed usually." The person put up for the murdered husband stands there, with no idea of what happened in the past, but then he falls to the floor. When someone asks, "What happened to you?" he answers, "I've been murdered." It just comes out of his mouth. Then the therapist asks if he wants to say anything to any of the other people. He speaks to his wife, and it becomes clear that she was the one who murdered him. They speak back and forth, and "very quickly, there's deep healing that happens between the two," states Dr. Klinghardt. "Usually we relive the pain and the truth that was there. . . . It's very, very dramatic. . . . Then the therapist does some healing therapeutic intervention with those representatives."

With removal of the interference that was transmitted down the generations, the client's condition is resolved, although the trickle-down effect to the lower levels of healing may need to be addressed. Often, however, healing at the higher level is sufficient. With balance restored at that level, the other levels are then able to correct themselves.

Dr. Klinghardt likens Family Systems Therapy to shamanic work in Africa, in which healing often has to be done from a distance through a representative because of the impracticability of a sick child, for example, traveling 200 miles from the village to see the medicine man. The representative holds a piece of clothing or hair from that child, and the shaman does the healing work on the stranger. "There's a magical effect broadcast back to the child," says Dr. Klinghardt. "The child often gets well. It's the same principle [with Family Systems Therapy]. We call it surrogate healing." He adds that Systemic Family Therapy has become very popular in Europe in the last two years, while it is still relatively new in the United States.

See Also For more about shamanic healing, see chapter 9.

Dr. Klinghardt has developed a variation of this technique that enables the work to happen with just a practitioner and the patient in a regular treatment room. He accomplishes the same end without representatives of the antecedents, using Autonomic Response Testing (ART, a kind of muscle testing; see "About the Therapies and Techniques") to pinpoint what happened and engage in the dialogues that arise in this work.

He gives the example of a 45-year-old woman who had lived

daily with asthma since she was two years old. Through ART, in a kind of process of elimination, Dr. Klinghardt learned that physical causes were not the source of the asthma and that it had to do with exclusion of some kind in a previous generation. Further exploration revealed that this woman's mother had lost a younger sibling when she was two years old. In this case, the woman knew of the event, but that was all she knew. ART confirmed the connection between this buried death and the asthma. Dr. Klinghardt stopped the session at this point, instructing his client to find out what she could about this family occurrence and then come back.

The woman's mother was still alive and told her that the baby died shortly after birth, was buried behind the house without a gravestone or other marker on the site, and was never mentioned again in the family. Everyone knew where the child was buried, but there was an unspoken agreement never to speak of her. Not only that, but the next child born was given the same name, as if the one who had died had never existed or, worse, had been replaced.

"This was a violation of a principle of what we know about Systemic Family Therapy, which is that each member who's born into a family has the same and equal right to belong to the family." Exclusion, even in memory, is a form of injustice and creates interference energy that is transmitted through the generations. Exclusion of a family member in the past is frequently the source of disturbance at the Intuitive Level, according to Dr. Klinghardt.

The client came back for the second session, and Dr. Klinghardt put her into a light trance state. "In that trance state she was able to contact that being, the dead sibling, and say to her, 'I remember you now, I bring you back into my family, I give you a place in my heart, I will never forget you.' Then she cried, and it was a very transformative experience." He observes that this process required very little guidance from him and took only about 20 minutes.

During the session, the woman made a commitment to go back to the house where the child was buried—it was still a family property—and put a gravestone on her grave. After the session, the woman's asthma was clearly better. She rated it at 50 to 60 percent better and reported later that it stayed that way. "It took her about three months to put up the gravestone, and she said the day after she set up the gravestone for that child, her asthma disappeared completely," relates Dr. Klinghardt. That was eight years ago, and the asthma has not returned.

Dr. Klinghardt and others who practice Family Systems Therapy have seen similar connections in cases of mental illness. Chronic anxiety or depression, schizophrenia, bipolar disorder, addiction, hyperactivity in children, aggressive behavior, and autism can all lead back to systemic family issues. In fact, Dr. Klinghardt estimates that "about 70 percent of mental disorders across the board go back to systemic family issues that need to be treated. People try to treat them psychologically, on the third level, and it cannot work. This is not the right level." Similarly, focusing on the biochemistry is not going to fix the problem when the source is at the fourth level.

The Fifth Level: The Spiritual

The fifth level is the direct relationship of the patient with God, or whatever name you choose for the divine. Interference in this relationship can be caused by early childhood experiences, past-life traumas, or enlightenment experiences with a guru or other spiritual teacher. Of the latter, Dr. Klinghardt says, "Some enlightenment experiences actually turn out to be a block. If the experience occurred in context with a guru, the person may become unable to reach enlightenment without the guru. The very thing that showed them what to look for becomes an obstacle."

This level requires self-healing when there is separation or interference in a person's connection to the divine. Direct contact with nature is one way to reforge the connection. "True prayer and true meditation work on this level as ways of getting there, but it's a level where there is no possibility of interaction between the healer and the patient," states Dr. Klinghardt. "I always say, if anybody tries to be helpful on this level, run as fast as you can." He notes that gurus and other spiritual teachers belong on the fourth level and have a valuable place there, but have no business on the fifth

Natural Medicine and the Five Levels of Healing

The chart below shows on what level the natural medicine therapeutic modalities in this book function.

Therapy	Level	Chapter
Applied Psychoneurobiology	Physical Body Electromagnetic Body Mental Body	3
CranioSacral Therapy	Physical Body Electromagnetic Body	7
Family Systems Therapy	Intuitive Body	3
Flower Essence Therapy	Mental Body	6
Homeopathy	Mental Body	5
NAET (allergy elimination)	Electromagnetic Body	3
Neural Therapy	Electromagnetic Body	3
Psychic/Shamanic Healing	Intuitive Body	9
Seemorg Matrix Work	Electromagnetic Body Mental Body	8
SomatoEmotional Release	Electromagnetic Body Mental Body	7
Thought Field Therapy	Electromagnetic Body Mental Body	3, 8
Traditional Chinese Medicine	Physical Body Electromagnetic Body	4
Visceral Manipulation	Physical Body Electromagnetic Body	7

level. If they trespass into that level, they are putting themselves where God should be, says Dr. Klinghardt. "It's very dangerous."

That said, a number of the therapies in this book clear impediments to spiritual connection at other levels, especially the Mental and Intuitive, thus opening the way for individuals to reestablish balance for themselves on the fifth level.

Operating Principles of the Five Healing Levels

The levels affect each other differently, depending on whether the influence is traveling upward or downward. Both trauma and successful therapeutic intervention at the higher levels have a rapid and deeply penetrating effect on the lower levels, says Dr. Klinghardt. This means that both the cause and the cure at the upper levels spread downward quickly. For example, if a systemic family issue is strongly present at the fourth (Intuitive) level, it will have profound effects on the first three levels. Similarly, resolving that issue can produce rapid changes in the Physical, Electromagnetic, and Mental Bodies. The lower levels may correct on their own, without further remediation.

At the same time, trauma or therapeutic intervention at the lower levels has a very slow and little penetrating effect upwards. When you get a physical injury (the first level), for instance, it will gradually change your electromagnetic field (the second level), altering the energy flow in your body. It's a slow process, however. The same is true for healing. "If you want to heal an injury on the second level, let's say you have a chakra that's blocked, you can do that by giving herbs and vitamins—biochemical interventions—but it will take years," says Dr. Klinghardt. But if you do an intervention on the third or fourth level, it can correct the blocked chakra on the second level immediately, within seconds or minutes, he notes.

Anxiety and the Five Levels of Healing

As stated earlier, anxiety can be the result of interference or disturbance on any of the Five Levels of Healing. In his practice, Dr. Klinghardt has discovered that the source of anxiety is most often found on the boundary between the second (Electromagnetic) and third (Mental) levels. Contribution on the second level often involves heavy metal toxicity. Allergies which, like heavy metals, create interference on both the Physical and Electromagnetic levels are also a common factor. Contribution on the third level "goes back to a traumatic event early in life," he explains.

Since Thought Field Therapy (TFT) operates on the very boundary where anxiety is most often found, it is a highly effective technique for eliminating the disorder. In fact, treating anxiety, phobia, and panic attacks is TFT's specialty. Unlike psychotherapy, which is an extended undertaking, the method is fast. "Anxiety is usually treated successfully with Thought Field Therapy, which takes less than five minutes to do in most people," observes Dr. Klinghardt. In his experience, about 90 percent of people suffering from anxiety respond with only one or two treatments.

Obsessive-compulsive disorder is slightly different. About 60 percent of cases respond to Thought Field Therapy, says Dr. Klinghardt. In these cases, the same mechanisms are in operation as with anxiety in general. For the other 40 percent, different causes are the source of the interference. "It can be on the fourth [Intuitive] level, but most commonly, it's a mineral disturbance on the first [Physical] level. With obsessive-compulsive disorder, you carefully look at the hair analysis, which shows the levels of minerals and heavy metals." Hair analysis is a laboratory test to determine the level of minerals and heavy metals in the hair, which is an indicator of the overall levels in the body.

For a more precise analysis of the body's level of heavy metals, Dr. Klinghardt injects the person with a chelating agent (DMPS), which will bind with heavy metals and carry them out of the body in the urine. (See Chelation in "About the Therapies and Techniques.") A urinalysis run after the chelating agent has had time to work then reveals what toxic metals are present in higher than normal levels in the body.

In the case of OCD, zinc deficiency or an inability to metabolize zinc properly is a common factor in the 40 percent who do not respond to Thought Field Therapy. If hair analysis indicates this may be a problem, Dr. Klinghardt may order a more precise test, a white blood cell zinc analysis, which looks at the zinc level inside the white blood cells. "Very often you find a deficiency there," he says, adding that "it's very difficult to raise these levels. You can't just give a zinc supplement and hope it's going to end up there. They can't absorb it, and they can't distribute it in the body properly."

Homeopathic zinc and intravenous zinc are two methods Dr. Klinghardt uses to get the levels up. He monitors the zinc levels for a few months, which is how long it generally takes for the body to take over and maintain the zinc level on its own. Manganese, both too much and too little, is another mineral factor that can be involved in OCD.

Mercury toxicity in the brain is a big factor in anxiety, as it is in depression. It and other types of heavy metal toxicity produce disturbances at both the Physical and Electromagnetic Levels, as explained previously. Chronic allergic reaction, another common factor, does the

In Their Own Words

"For me, a panic attack is almost a violent experience. I feel disconnected from reality. I feel like I'm losing control in a very extreme way. My heart pounds really hard, I feel like I can't get my breath, and there's an overwhelming feeling that things are crashing in on me."[150]
— a person with panic disorder

same. It keeps the immune system in an activated state, which weakens immunity (Physical), and the presence of allergenic substances disturbs the body's energy field (Electromagnetic).

Both heavy metal toxicity and allergies can prevent Thought Field Therapy from working. While the treatment may produce relief at first, it will not hold as it does with people for whom these factors are not an issue. In the case of allergies, the person is likely to relapse at the next exposure to an allergen. "With some people, it is newspaper print or car fumes. With others, it's eating a food that's toxic to them, that they're allergic to," Dr. Klinghardt notes.

To eliminate allergies, he uses NAET (see "About the Therapies and Techniques"). To get metals such as mercury out of the body, he relies on a method called oral chelation, using known natural chelators such as cilantro. He sometimes uses intravenous chelation with the amino acid glutathione, which is more aggressive in getting metals out of the brain.

As discussed previously, biophysical or geopathic stress amplifies the symptoms of heavy metal toxicity. Heavy metals are found mostly in the brain, where they work like antennae, Dr. Klinghardt elaborates. They pick up the electromagnetic or geopathic interference, which exacerbates anxiety and other symptoms.

For this reason, it may be important to consider the possibility of a contribution on the Electromagnetic Level in terms of sleeping location—the proximity of the bed to an electric outlet or positioning over a fault line or underground stream. If the anxiety is of recent onset, this is a factor to consider. Did the person recently move to a new home or change the position of the bed in the room? If the second level is involved in this way, simply changing the sleeping location can offer significant or complete relief.

Marta: Long-Term Anxiety Masking Depression

The following case history illustrates the relationship between anxiety and the levels of healing, and how the therapies Dr. Klinghardt uses remove these interferences and resolve even a seemingly intractable condition. This case also illustrates the close relationship between anxiety and depression, and how one can mask the other.

For eight years, Marta had been suffering from severe anxiety. She couldn't bear to be in a group of people, and, in fact, her anxiety had progressed to the point that she rarely left her house. She had been on the tranquilizer Xanax for quite some time and was worried about addiction to the medication. But whenever she tried to go off it, her anxiety got much worse. Recently, the Xanax had stopped working for her. She felt trapped; she had to find something else to keep her anxiety at bay, and yet she was afraid to go off the medication.

At this point, Marta sought the help of Dr. Klinghardt. His testing methods revealed that she was mercury toxic and had allergies to soybeans, wheat, and Xanax. It is common for people to develop an allergy to medications they take for a long time, says Dr. Klinghardt. "When you're allergic to something, there are two outcomes: you are miserable when you take it, or you become addicted to it." The latter was the case with Marta and her prescription drug.

To eliminate the mercury toxicity, Dr. Klinghardt started Marta on oral chelation, a program of oral supplements, such as the herb cilantro, known to function as chelators, or binding agents to remove heavy metals from the body. He notes that even if the source of the problem is on the fourth level, until you get the mercury out, Family Systems Therapy or other methods won't be able to clear the fourth-level interference. The mercury creates a kind of wall that prevents the other therapies from working. With the heavy metals removed, he has found that the psychological intervention can be accomplished in one to three sessions. In Marta's case, it was one, as you will see.

To address the allergies, he used an allergy clearing technique similar to NAET (see "About the Therapies and Techniques") to eliminate Marta's allergy to Xanax. In the case of wheat and soybeans, Marta opted to remove them from her diet. Immediately after the treatment, she started feeling better. She stayed on the Xanax and soon discovered that it worked once more like it had when she first started taking it.

She returned periodically for treatments to clear her other allergies and then decided she was ready to try to go off the Xanax, although it was still effective. For this, Dr. Klinghardt used Thought Field Therapy. He asked Marta to think about her anxiety in different situations while he used autonomic response testing (see "About the Therapies and Techniques") to determine which meridians went into a stress state. In her case, as is true of many people, the Spleen and Stomach meridians were the ones involved. Then he tapped gently with his fingertips on a series of points on these meridians, according to TFT patterns, while she again thought about the various situations that raised anxiety in her.

In most cases, it only takes one treatment with TFT to resolve anxiety, says Dr. Klinghardt. "You treat it once, and then it's gone forever." In Marta's case, it took two treatments because there was a situation she forgot to include the first time. She came back to get cleared on that one.

 For more about allergies, see chapter 2. For more about Thought Field Therapy, see chapter 8.

Then Dr. Klinghardt had Marta begin cutting down on the Xanax. Although she was no longer allergic to the medication, the drug is physiologically habit-forming, so withdrawal is a problem. To ease withdrawal symptoms, he gave her intravenous vitamin C and B vitamins twice a week for the three weeks of the weaning process. At the end of that period, she was off the drug and had made the transition without having to endure the withdrawal symptoms that usually attend such a process.

What happened then led to the revelation of the true source of her anxiety. With the anxiety peeled away, an underlying depression emerged. Marta told Dr. Klinghardt that it had always been there, but she had never focused on it. The anxiety had seemed more pressing, although in reality the depression was crippling her life as well.

Through Family Systems Therapy using ART, Marta connected the depression with her mother's sudden death in a car accident when Marta was 17. The way she dealt with that loss was to "march forward and try not to look back." Her operating principle became "Mom is gone, and I can do this on my own." It was at that point that her anxiety disorder began, with the ongoing depression beneath it.

Using Applied Psychoneurobiology, Dr. Klinghardt induced in Marta the mild hypnotic state that would allow her to go to the psychic level and reforge the link to her mother. After this experience, the depression disappeared and did not return. She also remained free of the anxiety that had plagued her for so long.

According to the tenets of Family Systems Therapy, Marta's refusal to grieve her mother's death was a kind of banishment of her mother from the family. It broke their psychic link and created a disturbance in Marta on the Intuitive Level, which manifested as depression. To remove the interference, she needed to reestablish the link with her mother. Using Applied Psychoneurobiology, Dr. Klinghardt induced in Marta the mild hypnotic state that would allow her to go to the psychic level and reforge the link to her mother. Through this process, Marta was able to recognize that her mother was always with her. After this experience, the depression disappeared and did not return. She also remained free of the anxiety that had plagued her for so long.

About the Therapies and Techniques

Applied Psychoneurobiology (APN): This therapeutic technique was developed by Dr. Klinghardt. Employing his muscle testing method (see ART below) as a guide, APN uses stress signals in the autonomic nervous system to communicate with a patient's unconscious mind. "You can establish a code with the unconscious mind for yes and no in answer to questions," he explains. "The code is the strength or the weakness of a test muscle." APN can lead the way to the beliefs that underlie disorders such as anxiety and exchange those beliefs with ones that promote balance in the Mental Body. This can produce dramatic shifts in the health and well-being of the person, notes Dr. Klinghardt.

Autonomic Response Testing (ART): ART, also called neural kinesiology, is a system of testing developed by Dr. Klinghardt. It employs a variety of methods, including muscle response testing and arm length testing, to measure changes in the autonomic nervous system. (The autonomic nervous system controls the automatic processes of the body such as respiration, heart rate, digestion, and response to stress.) ART is used to identify distress in the body and determine optimum treatment. In general, a strong arm (or finger, depending on the kind of muscle testing) or an even arm length (in arm length testing) indicates that the system is not in distress. A weak muscle or uneven arm length indicates the presence of a factor that is causing stress to the client's organism.

Chelation: This is a therapy that removes heavy metals from the body, among other therapeutic functions. DMPS (2,3-dimercaptopropane-1-sulfonate) is a substance used as a chelating agent, which means that it binds with heavy metals, notably mercury, and is then excreted from the body. DMPS can be administered orally, intravenously, or intramuscularly. Other chelation agents are cilantro, chlorella, alpha lipoic acid, and glutathione.

Nambudripad's Allergy Elimination Techniques (NAET):
NAET, developed by Devi S. Nambudripad, M.D., D.C., L.Ac.,
Ph.D., is a noninvasive and painless method for both identifying
and eliminating allergies. It uses kinesiology's muscle response testing to identify allergies. Chiropractic and acupuncture techniques
are then implemented to remove the energy blockages in the body
that underlie allergies, and to reprogram the brain and nervous system not to respond allergically to previously problem substances.

Neural Therapy: Developed by German physicians in 1925,
Neural Therapy employs the injection of local anesthetics (such as
procaine) or natural healing substances into specific sites in the
body to clear interferences in the flow of electrical energy and
restore proper nerve function. The interferences, or "interference
fields" as they are known in the profession, can be the result of a
scar, other old injury, physical trauma, or dental conditions such
as root-canaled or impacted teeth, all of which have their own
energy fields that can disrupt the body's normal energy flow.

Disruption in the body's energy field has far-flung effects and
can manifest in seemingly unrelated conditions. "Any part of the
body that has been traumatized or ill—no matter where it is
located—can become an interference field which may cause disturbance anywhere in the body," states Dr. Klinghardt.[151] Neural
therapy injections may be into glands, acupuncture points, or
ganglia (nerve bundles that are like relay stations for nerve
impulses), as well as scars or sites of trauma.

Thought Field Therapy (TFT): Psychotherapist Roger J.
Callahan, Ph.D., developed TFT in response to his frustration at
the failure of psychotherapy to help certain clients. It combines
principles of acupuncture and psychology to heal the Mental
Body. It actually operates on the boundary between the second
and third levels, the Electromagnetic and the Mental Bodies, says
Dr. Klinghardt. "The thought field is like a net that's attached on
the outside of the electromagnetic field. Through early childhood
trauma, the net is torn off the electric field." TFT restores the
attachment points between the electromagnetic and mental fields
and restores the proper energy flow in the body's meridians. It
accomplishes this through tapping gently with the fingertips on

certain points on the skin. These are acupuncture points that also correspond to the attachment sites, which are slightly out from the body. The tapping functions similarly to the needles in acupuncture, which remove energy blockages and restore the flow of energy along the meridians.

For more information about the therapies or to locate a practitioner near you, see the following:

- APN, ART, and Neural Therapy: Dr. Klinghardt (see appendix B); websites: www.neuraltherapy.com and www.pnf.org/neural_kinesiology.html.
- Chelation: The American College for Advancement in Medicine (ACAM), 23121 Verdugo Dr., Suite 204, Laguna Hills, CA 92653; fax: 949-455-9679; website: www.acam.org.
- NAET: Devi S. Nambudripad, M.D., D.C., L.Ac., Ph.D., Pain Clinic, 6714 Beach Blvd., Buena Park, CA 90621; tel: 714-523-8900; website: www.naet.com; also see her book *Say Good-Bye to Illness* (Buena Park, CA: Delta Publishing, 1999).
- TFT: *Tapping the Healer Within,* by Roger J. Callahan, Ph.D. (Chicago: Contemporary Books, 2001); for a practitioner, contact the Callahan Techniques office, 78-816 Via Carmel, La Quinta, CA 92253; tel: 760-564-1008; website: www.tftrx.com (professional site), www.selfhelpuniv.com (self-help site).

4 Energy Medicine I: Traditional Chinese Medicine

From the perspective of traditional Chinese medicine (TCM), any disorder, including anxiety, results from a disturbance in energy flow in the body. That disturbance produces effects in the person's mind and spirit as well as on the physical level because body, mind, and spirit are inseparable, says Ira J. Golchehreh, L.Ac., O.M.D., whose practice is based in San Rafael, California. All three operate on energy and are fed by the same source, so all three are affected when the energy becomes imbalanced. By restoring proper energy flow in the body, TCM treatment helps restore balance in mind and spirit as well as body.

Many people in the West do not understand that traditional Chinese medicine, of which acupuncture is a component, is a complex system and requires as rigorous, if not more rigorous, training as Western medicine in order to be practiced correctly. The programs at the better traditional Chinese medical schools take eight years to complete. Dr. Golchehreh is a master of TCM, having trained with professors from the Shanghai Medical School, which is considered the Harvard Medical School of Chinese medicine. He has treated tens of thousands of patients in the 20 years that he has been practicing and can reverse many intractable conditions that other forms of medicine have been unable to treat.

While every individual is unique, there are certain kinds of energy imbalances that typically accompany anxiety, Dr. Golchehreh says. Before we look at those patterns, let's get a better understanding of TCM and the energy it addresses.

What Is Traditional Chinese Medicine?

Traditional Chinese medicine was developed more than five thousand years ago in China and is still the predominant medical system used in that country today. It is also now widely practiced in the United States and other Western countries. The primary treatment modalities of TCM are acupuncture and Chinese herbal medicine. TCM is a form of energy, or vibrational, medicine, in that it is based on the flow of vital energy (*qi*, pronounced *chee*) in the body along energy channels known as meridians.

Another term for energy medicine is "molecular medicine," says Dr. Golchehreh. "When you look at the human being, you have to look at the molecular biology, the energy flow in the body, and the energy that is causing the vibrational weight between the cells and tissues."

Energy travels through the body along the meridians, which supply energy to organs, nerves, and other tissue. There are 12 primary meridians relating to the organs or organ systems, each bearing the name of the main organ it supplies, as in the Lung meridian, Heart meridian, Liver meridian, and Large Intestine meridian. In addition, there are two general meridians, the Governing Vessel and the Conception Vessel, as well as subsidiary energy channels.

Imbalances in energy flow can be excesses, deficiencies, or stagnation, and affect organs and systems throughout the body. TCM describes these imbalances and the attendant disharmony in the body in terms of natural world attributes such as heat, fire, cold, dampness, or dryness. These reflect the dominance of one or the other of the two essential qualities of *qi*: yin and yang. Yin is watery, dark, and calming, while yang is fiery, bright, and energizing. The names TCM uses to describe health conditions often have a poetic ring to them, as in Upflaming of Deficient Fire and Disorders of the Spirit Gate.

A doctor of Chinese medicine diagnoses the status of energy flow in a patient via the pulses, appearance of the tongue, and other physical and mien indications that practitioners are trained to observe. The pulses, though read at the wrist, are not the Western medicine pulse as in heart rate, but distinct pulses corresponding to the organs and meridians. The energy qualities of the various pulses are described in language such as wiry, thready, choppy, rapid, slow, floating, tight, and slippery. The quality signals to the practitioner the energy status of the organ and meridian.

As treatment, acupuncture and Chinese herbs are administered to address the specific energy imbalances of the patient: to raise deficient energy, reduce excess energy, or remove blockages producing energy stagnation.

In acupuncture, thin needles are shallowly inserted into the skin at strategic points (acupoints) along the meridian(s) requiring treatment, and left in place for an average of half an hour. This is a painless procedure, and patients often fall asleep while the needles are doing their work.

Acupuncture has application to a broad range of conditions but has become particularly known in the United States for its efficacy in relieving pain.

 In the United States, there are thousands of acupuncturists and doctors of traditional Chinese medicine. These medical practices require extensive training. Ask practitioners for information about their training and avoid those who have only taken a quick course. One organization that can help you locate an acupuncturist in your area is the National Certification Commission for Acupuncture and Oriental Medicine (NCCAOM), 11 Canal Center Plaza, Ste. 300, Alexandria, VA 22314; tel: 703-548-9004; website: www.nccaom.org.

Types of Anxiety in TCM

TCM divides anxiety into six classifications, according to symptoms and what is occurring in the energy meridians and the organs, as determined by TCM diagnosis, says Dr. Golchehreh.

They are 1) Mental Disturbance type; 2) Heart Blood Deficient type; 3) Excessive Deficient Fire type; 4) Heart Yang Deficient type; 5) Water (Fluid) Retention type; and 6) Blood Stasis type.

1. Mental Disturbance Type

The name of this category reflects the presenting symptoms, but the root of the disturbance is deficient energy on the Heart meridian. This type of anxiety is characterized by fearfulness. The person is easily frightened, by events and even by loud noises. The fear increases heart palpitations. Due to the fear level, insomnia is a problem in this type of anxiety. The tongue has a white coating. The pulses are very weak, but rapid.

You could also say of people with this type of anxiety that they are not strong enough mentally. This does not mean that they are not intelligent. The mind and heart are closely connected energetically, says Dr. Golchehreh. "People who have heart disease, for example, get forgetful; the mind cannot concentrate. You get symptoms of forgetfulness with malfunction of the heart. This is because the Heart meridian controls the nervous system, which controls the mind." The fact that heart palpitations typically accompany an anxiety attack supports the Chinese medicine view that anxiety reflects a problem on the Heart meridian.

An energy imbalance in the Heart meridian can throw off the balance of neurotransmitters in the brain, notes Dr. Golchehreh. Proper chemistry can be restored by restoring the function of the Heart meridian. This relationship explains why psychiatric medications that attempt to manipulate the biochemistry of the brain do not solve the problem: antianxiety drugs do not address the root energy problem that threw the biochemistry out of balance in the first place.

Treatment for the Mental Disturbance type of anxiety involves acupuncture and Chinese herbs aimed at "tonifying the heart and soothing the unstable mind," Dr. Golchehreh says. This means strengthening or supporting the function of the heart and stabilizing or calming the mind. The acupuncturist accomplishes this by working on the Pericardium channel rather than directly on the Heart meridian. The reason for this it that it is not the heart itself that is producing the palpitations associated with

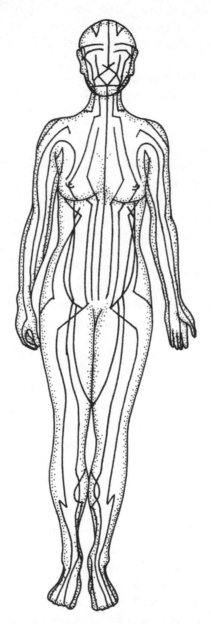

Acupuncture Meridians

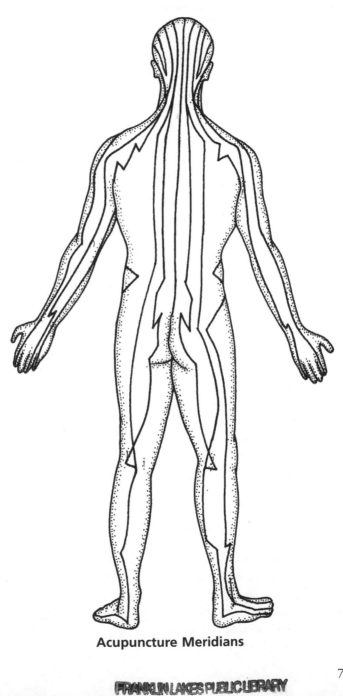

Acupuncture Meridians

anxiety, but rather the pericardium (membranous sac around the heart) clenching around the heart and causing spasms. By calming the Pericardium channel, the heart is calmed.

Acupuncture treatment of a meridian has far-reaching effects. "It is important to remember," says Dr. Golchehreh, "that when we're treating the Heart (Pericardium) meridian, it is not only the meridian, but all of the nerves that are supplied by that meridian. It's a network of the nervous system, which carries the biochemistry that is behind the function of that organ." Further, while the central problem may be on one meridian, acupuncture treatment will likely include other meridians as well, because an imbalance in one meridian produces energy flow problems in others.

The goal of strengthening the heart and calming the mind is "to get the heart back in charge, controlling the mind." The herbs that help with this are a licorice and jujube combination. "These are the herbs traditionally used in Chinese medicine to tonify the heart and smooth the unstable mind," Dr. Golchehreh explains.

2. Heart Blood Deficient Type

The Heart Blood Deficient type of anxiety is similar to the Mental Disturbance type, but the primary symptoms, aside from the palpitations, are poor memory, great fatigue, and paleness. "These people don't have any color," says Dr. Golchehreh, which is a sign of compromised heart function. This type usually involves a deficiency on the Spleen meridian as well. "Since the heart is not pumping the blood correctly, and the spleen is not providing the heart with the blood that it needs, it causes fatigue, low energy." In these cases, the tongue is red and may not have any coating. The pulses are thready, weak, and thin.

Treatment focuses on tonifying or strengthening the heart and the spleen. "Since the spleen provides the blood and the heart provides the *qi*, strengthening the heart and the spleen makes the *qi* and the blood strong," explains Dr. Golchehreh. Acupuncture treats the Heart and Spleen meridians to correct the deficient energy flow. The herbs used are those known to strengthen the heart, spleen, and *qi*. A ginseng and longan combination is a good one for this, according to Dr. Golchehreh.

3. Excessive Deficient Fire Type

The primary symptoms of this type are breathlessness and dizziness because of the deficiency. The excessive deficient fire aspect results in heart palpitations, sleep problems, high restlessness, and quickness to anger. "The fire types have the sensation of heat in the body. You can feel the heat coming out of their hands and the bottom of their feet." In addition, the lumbar region of the back becomes weak and sore; in the female, menstruation becomes very irregular. The tongue is red. The pulses are rapid and thready.

Excessive and deficient seem to be contradictory, but Dr. Golchehreh explains the condition in this way: "If the energy is deficient, it should not be coming up. But when there is fire, it means the yin is depleted." (Remember that all energy has complementary yin and yang aspects.) "With the yin depleted, the yang is in excess. The yang, or fire, is allowed to come to the surface. The yin is like water to the system. When we have a deficient yin, there's no cooling effect and it causes the fire to upflame." Thus, Excessive Deficient Fire (excess fire born of deficient yin).

To treat this condition, it is necessary to tonify (strengthen) the yin, to bring up the water to cool down the fire, so to speak. In this type of anxiety, the Kidney meridian is the site of the deficient yin—in TCM, the kidneys are considered to hold the essence of life—so it is the focus of acupuncture treatment. Acupuncture and herbs work together to tonify the yin, clear the heat (the excess yang), and tranquilize the mind. Indicated herbs for this are lycium, chrysanthemum, and rehmannia.

4. Heart Yang Deficient Type

With this type of anxiety, people have a "continuous, uncontrollable, violent throbbing of the heart. In other words, the heart is pumping very hard and fast," says Dr. Golchehreh, adding that it feels like you are having a heart attack. Without the action of the yang (fire) to control the yin, the latter is like floodwater rising in a river and overflowing the banks. "This causes the heart to be in a throbbing state, with uncontrolled movement pushing through the heart valves, heart muscles, and the entire system, producing a suffocating sensation in the chest."

TCM Types of Anxiety

1. Mental Disturbance Type

Symptoms: Fearfulness, heart palpitations, insomnia
Pulses: Very weak, but rapid
Tongue: White coating
Primary meridian(s) involved: Pericardium
Treatment: Tonify the heart, smooth the unstable mind
Herbs: Licorice, jujube

2. Heart Blood Deficient Type

Symptoms: Heart palpitations, poor memory, fatigue, paleness
Pulses: Thready, weak, and thin
Tongue: Red and may not have a coating
Primary meridian(s) involved: Heart and Spleen
Treatment: Tonify the heart and spleen
Herbs: Ginseng, longan

3. Excessive Deficient Fire Type

Symptoms: Dizziness, heart palpitations, sleep problems, high restlessness, quickness to anger, weak and sore lower back, irregular menstruation, feeling of heat in the body
Pulses: Rapid and thready
Tongue: Red
Primary meridian(s) involved: Kidney
Treatment: Tonify the yin, clear the heat, tranquilize the mind
Herbs: Lycium, chrysanthemum, rehmannia

4. Heart Yang Deficient Type

Symptoms: Continuous, uncontrollable, violent throbbing of the heart, shortness of breath, pain may radiate to the right shoulder and right side of the neck, cold extremities
Pulse: Very weak, no force
Tongue: Pale
Primary meridian(s) involved: Heart
Treatment: Warm and tonify the heart yang, calm the disturbed mind
Herbs: Cinnamon and dragon bone combination; cinnamon, atractylodes, and aconite combination

5. Water (Fluid) Retention Type

Symptoms: Heart palpitations, dizziness, feeling of fullness in the chest, water retention (edema), especially in the lower body, cold extremities, reduced or dribbling urination, thirst but no desire to drink, nauseous upon drinking water

Pulse: Wiry and slippery

Tongue: Smooth, white

Primary meridian(s) involved: Kidney

Treatment: Strengthen the kidney yang to promote the *qi* and water circulation

Herbs: Hoelen and atractylodes combination; bupleurum, cinnamon, and ginger combination

6. Blood Stasis Type

Symptoms: Heart palpitations, listlessness, restlessness, suffocating sensation in the chest, general chest pain, purplish hue to fingernails

Pulse: Rocky

Tongue: Dark, purplish

Primary meridian(s) involved: Pericardium and Heart

Treatment: Regulate the *qi* and promote blood circulation

Herbs: Tang-Kuei Four combination, carthmus, and persica seed

This puts pressure on the lungs which, in turn, causes shortness of breath; difficulty taking a deep breath. With increasing yin in the chest, pain and discomfort can radiate to the right shoulder and right side of the neck. Dr. Golchehreh notes that this is in contrast to the radiating pain on the left side during a heart attack. Yang deficiency, as in this case, produces effects on the right side, while yin deficiency produces effects on the left side.

In the Heart Yang Deficient type of anxiety, the limbs and extremities are cold, because yin is cold. Yin is also pale, so the tongue is always pale in these cases, says Dr. Golchehreh. The pulses have no force.

Treatment focuses on warming and tonifying the heart yang (which means strengthening it to bring up the natural heat of yang) and calming the disturbed mind by restoring proper energy balance on the Heart meridian and giving herbs that have these effects. Particularly helpful herbs are a combination of cinnamon and dragon bone, and a combination of cinnamon, atractylodes, and aconite.

5. Water (Fluid) Retention Type

In this type, it is fluid in the heart that is causing the problem. As with all other types of anxiety, heart palpitations are part of the symptom picture, as are dizziness and a feeling of fullness in the chest. "The chest feels like it is filled with fluid," Dr. Golchehreh explains. The whole body is filled with fluid, due to water retention (edema). This is especially evident in the lower body, as an effect of gravity.

As water is cold by nature, the extremities are cold. People with this type of anxiety don't urinate as much as normal (dribbling urination is characteristic) because the body is retaining fluid. At the same time, they feel thirsty, but have no desire to drink. When they do, they will become nauseated and feel like vomiting. The tongue typically has a smooth white appearance. The pulses are wiry and slippery, like water.

To reverse this watery state, it is necessary to bring up or strengthen the kidney yang (the energy of heat to dry out some of the water), which promotes both the *qi* and water circulation. Acupuncture treatment accomplishes this by focusing on restoring the proper flow of energy on the Kidney meridian. Herbal medicines indicated for this condition are a combination of hoelen and atractylodes, and a combination of bupleurum, cinnamon, and ginger, all of which work to strengthen the kidney yang.

6. Blood Stasis Type

With this type, people have heart palpitations because the blood is not moving smoothly. The blood stagnation causes them to feel both listless and restless. "If the blood doesn't get smoothly to the heart, it causes restlessness," Dr. Golchehreh explains. The stagnation also produces a suffocating sensation in the chest, as though the chest were full, similar to what people experience in the Heart Yang Deficient type of anxiety. Again, they may think they are having a heart attack, but in this case, the pain is all over the chest.

In addition, the fingernails have a purplish hue underneath instead of the normal red hue because the blood has lost its healthy red tone due to congestion. "The same quality shows on the tongue," notes Dr. Golchehreh. "It's darkish instead of clear and red." The pulse is typically rocky, "like a rock moving under your finger," the opposite of the slippery watery feeling of the Water Retention type.

Treatment is aimed at regulating the *qi* and promoting blood circulation to get the blood moving again. For this, the focus is on the Pericardium and Heart meridians, and acupuncture points that specifically address the blood, called general blood points. The herbal medicines that Dr. Golchehreh uses to regulate the *qi* and break down blockage to get the blood circulating again are Tang-Kuei Four combination, carthmus, and persica seed. Persica seed clears the function of the small intestines, which is related to and therefore has an impact on heart function, he explains.

> **Genetics may be a factor. You can inherit a tendency for your qi to be deficient (or in excess), Dr. Golchehreh notes. "That genetic tendency could go back centuries." This inheritance can set you up for anxiety.**

Causes of Energy Disturbance

The flow of vital energy (*qi*) in the body can be thrown out of balance—become excessive, deficient, blocked, or stagnant— by influences on the physical, psychological, or spiritual levels. Biochemical, functional, or metabolic factors can be involved. A poor diet, organ malfunction, toxicity, and stress all affect energy flow in the body. It is the chicken or the egg issue, however. For example, did a psychological trauma disrupt the flow of *qi*, which in turn threw off the body's biochemistry? Or did a poor diet result in biochemical deficiencies, which led to energy disturbance and psychological problems?

Genetics may be a factor as well. You can inherit a tendency for your *qi* to be deficient (or in excess), Dr. Golchehreh notes. "That genetic tendency could go back centuries." This inheritance can set you up for anxiety.

The factors that affect *qi* can be internal or external. Just as the body, mind, and spirit are related within a human being, human beings are also elements in the environment, he states. "You're definitely under the influence of what's going on outside, physically, chemically, and in every other way. Your body chemistry has a tendency to fluctuate accordingly. We are not individual parts. We are a part of the whole. That's why the pollution in the air, for example, could also cause some kind of problems internally, like in the lung, the heart, and the liver."

In acupuncture, as with other natural medicine modalities, there are layers of healing. Underneath the energy imbalances that are producing the presenting symptoms may be other energy imbalances that can be addressed once the "top" layer is removed, explains Dr. Golchehreh. What is presenting on top is the acute aspect, and what is underlying is the chronic. "So there are different layers of a problem that affect a person psychologically, mentally, and physically," he concludes.

The complexity of influences involved in "mental" disorders such as anxiety makes it imperative to consider the person as a whole—body, mind, and spirit—in treatment, as TCM does. "You cannot just give them a drug and send them home," says Dr. Golchehreh.

Jim: Courtroom Anxiety

Jim, 39, was a successful defense attorney. For many years, he had suffered from anxiety attacks, often in the courtroom, but the attacks were increasing in severity. Actually, they would begin the night before a court appearance when he would be unable to sleep without the aid of a strong sleeping pill. The next day in court, he would have heart palpitations and stabbing chest pains, his palms would become hot and sweaty, his back and shoulders would stiffen so severely as to produce pain, and his speech would start to slur.

During his anxiety attacks, Jim felt like he was having a heart attack and had ended up in the emergency room on more than one occasion. He sought the help of a cardiologist, who could find nothing organically wrong. His EKG (electrocardiogram) was normal, his blood pressure was normal, and he was in good physical shape.

So far, Jim had been able to hide his attacks in the courtroom, but he was afraid that they would get to the point where he could no longer conceal what was happening to him. The slurred speech was especially worrisome in this regard. It was at this juncture that he sought the help of Dr. Golchehreh.

Having listened to Jim's heart and taken his blood pressure to confirm that they were normal, Dr. Golchehreh's next step was to take his pulses while asking him questions about the anxiety attacks: when they occurred, how often, what happened during them. While talking about the attacks, Jim's pulses, which had previously been calm, became very rapid. "When you ask a question that relates to the cause of the problem, the quality of the pulse changes," Dr. Golchehreh observes. This is a means of pinpointing the source of the disorder. It also supported the evidence that a heart problem was not operational in Jim's case.

Dr. Golchehreh determined that Jim's anxiety was of the Excessive Deficient Fire type, as evidenced by his red tongue, rapid and thready pulses, and other symptoms. "The heart is where the soul and the spirit are centered, and when they are disturbed, it causes disharmony in other parts of the body, affecting all the other organs' functions." In Jim's case, all of his organs had

> ## In Their Own Words
>
> *"I awoke one night out of a sound sleep with a racing, irregular heartbeat, difficulty breathing, and an incredible feeling of terror. I was 27 then, and it was my first panic attack."*[152]
>
> —a woman whose panic attacks led to agoraphobia

deficient energy, but at the same time he was "fire-ish," as characterizes this type of deficiency syndrome in Chinese medicine.

To treat him, Dr. Golchehreh used acupuncture on points on the Pericardium channel to calm the soul and spirit. "By doing that, you not only treat the heart and the pericardium, you actually calm the soul and spirit of the *qi* and blood, which goes through all the other organs of the body." He also treated points on the Kidney meridian, as is indicated for this type of anxiety. For Chinese herbal medicine, in Jim's case he got ginseng to strengthen him because he was so deficient and zizyphus, which calms the spirit. It is important to note here that, while certain treatments tend to go with the different types of anxiety, there is no standard treatment in traditional Chinese medicine. The specifics of treatment are tailored to the individual.

The acupuncture and herbs worked together to tonify the yin, clear the heat, and tranquilize the mind and in the process restore the energy balance in Jim's body. The first few sessions didn't produce much of a difference, which was to be expected, according to Dr. Golchehreh. After the readjustment effected through acupuncture, "it takes a little bit of time for the organs to go back to normal functioning," he says. This is especially true in chronic cases.

After three weeks of twice-weekly acupuncture treatments, however, Jim's symptoms were nearly gone. He was no longer having anxiety attacks, though he had been in the courtroom numerous times during that period. His speech would still slur on occasion, though.

In looking at the psychological aspect of his anxiety attacks, Jim made the connection that the attacks had begun when he began to practice as an attorney. With further exploration, he realized that the attacks came when he was handling a case in which he knew the client was lying to him and was probably guilty as charged, despite the client's protestations to the contrary. His anxiety attacks reflected his internal conflict over defending a lying, guilty client. In this light, his slurred speech could be seen as representative of a moral reluctance to use his powers of speech to get the guilty party off.

This is not an irreconcilable situation, according to Dr. Golchehreh. In such cases, he teaches his patients to take deep breaths, calm the mind, and relax the body before entering the conflictual situation (the courtroom, in Jim's case). Meditation is also a good protective measure. Keeping the energy flowing properly in the body is another important preventive tool. When there is energy disturbance, psychological conflicts can much more easily throw us off. Another way to say it is that energy disturbances leave us much more vulnerable to stress.

In energetic terms, Jim's psychological conflict contributed to creating the energy disturbances in his body, and then those energy disturbances in turn compounded his reaction to the conflict. With the body in balance, we are better able to meet problematic situations.

This was the case with Jim. It has been three years since he had an anxiety attack. Having learned the importance of balanced energy flow, he periodically comes back to Dr. Golchehreh for a "tune-up." The last time was when he was representing someone he was "not too happy about." In this way, he is able to continue the work to which he is dedicated and at the same time prevent a return of the energy imbalance and anxiety attacks that made his life so difficult.

5 Energy Medicine II: Homeopathy

In addition to acupuncture, another form of energy medicine is particularly effective in the treatment of anxiety: homeopathy. Homeopathy is similar to flower essence therapy (see next chapter) in that the medicines they employ do not contain biochemical components of the plants (or other substances, in the case of homeopathy) from which they are derived, but transfer their energetic patterns. The medicines help restore the individual's energy (or vital force, or *qi*) to its natural equilibrium and thus return balance to the body, mind, and spirit.

Judyth Reichenberg-Ullman, N.D., L.C.S.W., of Edmonds, Washington, is an internationally known naturopathic and homeopathic physician. She and her husband, Robert Ullman, N.D., teach, lecture, and have written numerous books together, including *Prozac Free: Homeopathic Alternatives to Conventional Drug Therapies.* Their column on homeopathic treatment has run in the esteemed journal *Townsend Letter for Doctors and Patients* since 1990.

Dr. Reichenberg-Ullman went into homeopathy because of her interest in mental health. In her early career as a psychiatric social worker, she worked on a locked psychiatric ward, in emergency rooms, nursing homes, halfway houses, and patients' homes. "I saw the whole spectrum of mental illness, and the suffering was terrible," she recalls. "I didn't see conventional medicine as having a magic bullet for most of these people. With the degree of side effects they were experiencing [from medications], I thought there must be something better."

Dr. Reichenberg-Ullman discovered that "something better" in homeopathy, as did her husband. They wrote *Prozac Free* to share their discovery of an effective alternative to medications for anxiety, depression, and other psychiatric disorders. "As shown by the numerous patients we have treated successfully, we believe we have found a method that can transform the lives of many people," she states.[153] "Homeopathy can't help everybody, but the number of people that can be helped with these impairing mental and emotional conditions is incredibly gratifying."

As a treatment for anxiety, homeopathy is not only "safe, long-lasting, and highly effective," she says, but it also "has the potential to alleviate your physical problems as well."[154] This is because homeopathy addresses the underlying imbalance that is responsible for all of a person's symptoms. The imbalance occurs on an energetic level, which is why an energy medicine such as homeopathy is so effective in restoring balance. Let's look more closely at the concept of energy imbalance.

We are energetic organisms, or energy-modulated organisms, explains Dr. Reichenberg-Ullman, and that energy is our vital force or *qi*, as it is known in traditional Chinese medicine. "The vital force of each person has a certain susceptibility. Due to that susceptibility, there are going to be certain factors that trigger an imbalance or symptoms in that person."

For example, in a family in which one parent has bipolar disorder (the mood disorder formerly known as manic-depression), which research has shown to have a genetic component, one of the children develops the illness and the others don't. That one child was susceptible in some way. The same is true of nonpsychiatric illnesses, Dr. Reichenberg-Ullman points out, citing epidemics as an example. Even in virulent epidemics, there are people who are not susceptible and do not contract the illness, she notes.

In homeopathic terms, susceptibility relates to the state of a person's vital force. "It's important to realize that the vital force or the energetic equilibrium of that individual is the bottom line," says Dr. Reichenberg-Ullman. "When there is an imbalance, a disturbance underneath the surface of the lake, then there are ripples that go out. Those ripples can manifest in any number of ways." Anxiety can be one of those manifestations.

Scientific consensus currently holds that neurotransmitter problems are the factor behind mental disorders. In actuality, the research supporting this is "still more theoretical than they would make it out to be," says Dr. Reichenberg-Ullman. In her view, a deeper imbalance in a person's energetic equilibrium is what throws neurotransmitter supply and function out of balance.

Thus, simply attempting to control brain biochemistry is not getting to the real source of the mental disorder. "You have to deal with that underlying disturbance, or else it's like putting your finger in the dike, which I think is what, to a large degree, conventional medicine is doing," Dr. Reichenberg-Ullman states. The rampant prescription of antianxiety and antidepressant medications to both adults and children to deal with the epidemic of anxiety and depression in the United States and other developed countries is a prime example of the finger in the dike.

Dr. Reichenberg-Ullman cites a cultural component as a factor in anxiety. "Certain cultures tend to be more relaxed. But in others, like our culture, like Japan probably, where there's so much pressure, I think that fosters a lot more anxiety. There is a cultural overstimulation and obsessiveness."

Environmental factors such as these or traumatic life events can have an impact on your vital force. Grief over the death of a loved one, for example, weakens your vital force and leaves you susceptible to the ripple effect of an energy imbalance. Homeopathy can provide support at these times and serve as an intervention that keeps the cycle from escalating. Dr. Reichenberg-Ullman recalls her days of ministering to people whose family members died in the emergency room. "The psychiatric social workers are wonderful, but all they have to offer are antianxiety medications like Xanax," she notes. "If there were someone there offering homeopathy as one of the alternatives, it would be of great benefit."

Homeopathy can restore balance thrown off by what Dr. Reichenberg-Ullman calls the tumults or turmoils of life. Psychotherapy, while providing important tools and support, does not necessarily address the vital force disequilibrium caused by these tumults. People who have been through a challenging event or are in a difficult life situation may, despite therapy, still have a lot of fear and not feel in control of their lives. "Homeopathy can bring them into balance in a way that they didn't think was possible," she states.

Like many natural medicine physicians, Dr. Reichenberg-Ullman re-

gards symptoms, whether mental, emotional, or physical, as an individual's attempt to cope with the underlying disturbance. The body has its own wisdom, and symptoms are the ways in which a particular person adapts to the imbalance in their vital force. The beauty of homeopathy is that it goes to the heart of the matter and corrects the disturbance in the vital force. From that, all the other imbalances correct as well. This is why homeopathy can address both your anxiety and whatever physical problems you are manifesting.

What Is Homeopathy?

To understand homeopathy, it is helpful to consider the derivation of the word as well as that of allopathy, both of which were coined by the father of homeopathy, Dr. Samuel Hahnemann, in the late 1700s. A German physician and chemist who became increasingly frustrated with conventional medical practice, Dr. Hahnemann devoted himself to developing a safer, more effective approach to medicine. The result was homeopathy, which arose out of his discovery that illness can be treated by giving the patient a dilution of a plant that produces symptoms resembling those of the illness when given to a healthy person.

This principle, "let likes be cured with likes," became known as the Law of Similars. Dr. Hahnemann named this system of healing "homeopathy," a combination of the Greek *homoios* (similar) and *pathos* (suffering). At the same time, he dubbed conventional medicine "allopathy," which means "opposite suffering," to reflect that model's approach of treating illness by giving an antidote to the symptoms, a medicine that produces the opposite effect from what the patient is suffering. (A laxative for constipation is an illustration of the allopathic approach; it produces diarrhea.)[156]

Homeopathic remedies can be employed as a simple remedy to address a certain transitory ailment or as a constitutional remedy to address the more permanent constellation of physical, psychological, and emotional characteristics—the constitution—of an individual patient. A constitutional remedy works to restore balance and thus health on all levels.

Homeopathic remedies are prepared through a process of dilution of plant, mineral, or animal substances, which results in a "potentized" remedy, one that contains the energy imprint of the substance rather than its biochemical components. This is why homeopathy falls into the category of energy medicine; it works on an energetic level to effect change in all aspects of a person and restore balance to the whole.

Paradoxically, the higher the number of dilutions, the greater the potency and the effects of the remedy. Thus the higher the potency number, the more powerful the remedy. Remedies used to treat a transitory condition are usually 6C, 12C, or 30C, relatively low-potency remedies. A constitutional remedy is often a 200C potency, which means it has been diluted 200 times (99 parts alcohol or water to one part substance), or a 1M potency, which means it has been diluted a thousand times.

Constitutional Treatment of Anxiety

Classical or constitutional homeopathic treatment is distinct from the use of homeopathic remedies for acute symptoms in that it employs a single remedy that addresses the particular and unique mental, emotional, and physical state of an individual. Dr. Reichenberg-Ullman explains it this way: "Each child, or adult, is much like a jigsaw puzzle. Once all of the pieces are assembled in their proper places, an image emerges that is distinct from other puzzles. It is the task of a homeopath to recognize that image and to match it to the corresponding image of one specific homeopathic medicine."[157]

The homeopath makes that match by considering the person's behaviors, feelings, attitudes, beliefs, likes, dislikes, physical symptoms, prenatal and birth history, family medical history, eating and sleeping patterns, and even dreams and fears.[158] By giving the remedy whose qualities match this unique cluster most closely, the homeopathic principle of "like cures like" is put into operation, and the remedy works to restore the person to balance.

Homeopathy does not prescribe according to diagnostic labels, but rather according to the complete picture of the individual. Thus, there is no universal remedy for anxiety, and two people suffering from it will likely require two entirely different remedies, chosen from more than two thousand possible homeopathic remedies.

People may have one constitutional remedy that is their match throughout their life, or they may change over time and a different constitutional remedy might then be required.

Homeopathy does not prescribe according to diagnostic labels, but rather according to the complete picture of the individual. Thus, there is no universal remedy for anxiety, and two people suffering from it will likely require two entirely different remedies, chosen from more than two thousand possible homeopathic remedies.

It's interesting to note that the qualities of the remedy that is the correct one for a person reflect their areas of susceptibility or vulnerability. "When a certain homeopathic medicine benefits a person, that tells me something about that person," observes Dr.

Reichenberg-Ullman. "From understanding that homeopathic medicine, I know what kinds of conditions, whether mental, emotional, or physical, that the person is likely to be susceptible to and what kinds they aren't. It often gives you a predictive capacity. Conventional medicine doesn't understand people deeply enough in most cases to be able to do that."

A single dose of a constitutional remedy is often all that is needed at first (though the remedy may also be given more often, even daily). When the remedy is the correct one for an individual, changes can begin relatively quickly, within one to five weeks after taking the dose. (Some people experience changes in the first day, or even within hours.) If there are no changes within five weeks, that generally indicates that it is not the proper remedy. A remedy continues to work over time, anywhere from four months to a year or longer. Repeat doses may be necessary if there is a relapse of symptoms, or sometimes a different remedy may be called for.

Due to the way homeopathic remedies work, it is important to continue treatment for one to two years at least, states Dr. Reichenberg-Ullman. This does not necessarily entail frequent appointments with your homeopath, however. As stated, a single dose of a remedy works for some time.

While certain substances (notably coffee, menthol, camphor, and eucalyptus) can antidote single-dose homeopathic remedies in some sensitive individuals, prescription medications may not interfere with their function. Topical steroids, antibiotics, and antifungals and oral antibiotics and cortisone products may act suppressively and are best used in consultation with your homeopath.[159] Be assured, however, that homeopathic remedies do not interfere with the function of conventional medicine. Thus, you can pursue homeopathic treatment while continuing your medications or working with your prescribing doctor to phase them out when possible.

As a final note, regarding the efficacy of homeopathy in treating panic attacks, Dr. Reichenberg-Ullman states, "Homeopathic effectiveness is most limited by the skill, knowledge, and experience of the homeopath and the cooperation of the patient. The theory works, but it must be applied well and for a long enough time with sufficient expertise to produce results."[160]

 There are more than one thousand classical homeopaths in the United States, a small percentage of whom specialize in mental health. One source to help you find a qualified homeopath in your area is the Homeopathic Academy of Naturopathic Physicians (HANP), 1412 W. Washington St., Boise, ID 83702; tel: 208-336-3390; website: www.hanp.org.

Sally: Panic Attacks and Multiplying Fears

This case from the patient files of Dr. Reichenberg-Ullman illustrates how homeopathy can significantly help individuals suffering from panic attacks and debilitating fear.*

When Sally, 34, came to Dr. Reichenberg-Ullman, she was suffering from increasingly severe panic attacks and a growing number of fears that left her in sheer terror.

A primary fear was of flying. Originally from England, she had flown back and forth across the Atlantic many times, but her fear of flying had increased over the last several years to the point of panic attacks. During these, she experienced extreme anxiety and violent heart palpitations, which felt as though her heart were going to leap out of her chest. She was terrified because she knew that the plane would crash—knew that something was wrong and it was only a matter of time before they went down. Her anxiety increased with any in-flight turbulence or when the seatbelt sign remained on past the point when she thought it would normally be turned off. "The only way she could become calm was to

---

*This case study adapted, by permission of Judyth Reichenberg-Ullman, N.D., L.C.S.W., from her book, written with Robert Ullman, N.D., *Prozac Free: Homeopathic Alternatives to Conventional Drug Therapies* (Berkeley, CA: North Atlantic Books, 2002), pages 122-125.

The Benefits of Homeopathic Treatment

Dr. Reichenberg-Ullman cites the following benefits of constitutional homeopathic treatment.[161] Homeopathy

- treats the whole person

- treats the root of the problem

- treats each person as an individual

- uses natural, nontoxic medicines

- is considered safe and does not have the side effects of prescription drugs

- heals physical, mental, and emotional symptoms

- uses medicines, one dose of which works for months or years rather than hours

- uses inexpensive medicines

- is cost effective

remind herself that she had absolutely no control over the situation," recalls Dr. Reichenberg-Ullman.

Sally's fear of flying had become particularly severe the year before, after she learned that the child she was carrying, her first, was dead. She shook all night before the stillbirth delivery, which was scheduled for the next day. The recurrent shaking fits she had after that became paired in her mind with transatlantic flight.

Another fear occurred for Sally whenever she drove across a bridge. Before the stillbirth, she had felt panic, imagining the car going off the side into the water below, but she was able to put those thoughts out of her mind. After the death of her daughter, however, she was compelled to play out the whole scene whenever she crossed a bridge, picturing the car going into the water, her vain struggle to open the doors, then trying to open the windows and save her husband and herself. Terror flooded her at these times at the thought that they might not be able to escape and she might make the wrong decision, leading to one or both of them drowning. She experienced the panic attack whether she was driving or in the passenger seat.

Other fears developed, all with a disaster scenario. When she stayed in a hotel, she became anxious that there was going to be a devastating fire. She worried about having a heart attack, breast cancer, or other serious health problem. Since the doctors had been unable to tell her why her infant had died in the womb, she might have something very wrong with her that doctors had missed. She was fearful, too, that she, like one of her family's friends, might die during childbirth in the future. In summary, she felt an extreme fear of mortality.

Fear was not a new phenomenon for Sally. Despite her happy childhood in rural England, she had always been a worrier. Now, however, the fears had multiplied and were far more serious. At times, her anxiety would wake her every hour throughout the night. She worried that something horrible would befall her husband. A sound in the night could send her into a panic that someone was breaking into the house and was going to kill them. As on the plane and the bridge, she would play out the scenario in her mind, from running to the phone and calling 911 to escaping out the door.

"My imagination just goes wild. I tend to take little things and blow them way out of proportion," Sally told Dr. Reichenberg-Ullman. During their initial consultation, it also emerged that a deep sense of failure had plagued Sally since the death of her child. Being a mother was what she had envisioned for herself, and she hadn't been able to make it happen. "She lived in fear of others asking her if she had any children," says Dr. Reichenberg-Ullman.

The physical problems Sally reported were periodic rashes and herpes on her face, heavier and longer menstrual periods with a lot of clotting, and a persistent vaginal discharge.

The constitutional remedy for Sally was *Argentum nitricum* (silver nitrate). "This is a medicine for people with anticipatory anxiety of all kinds," explains Dr. Reichenberg-Ullman. "They often have claustrophobia and a fear of heights and bridges. Those needing this medicine have a perpetual tendency to imagine disasters and catastrophes, and therefore are likely candidates for phobias and panic attacks."

Five weeks later, Sally reported that her anxiety over flying was much less. In fact, she had flown from the West Coast to Chicago with no problems. She no longer ran the scenario about driving off a bridge. The heart palpitations were gone, and she was sleeping better.

At that point, she also reported a patch of ringworm (a skin rash), which she had not had for 20 years, but had frequently as a child. This was nothing to be alarmed about, and was actually part of Sally's healing response, Dr. Reichenberg-Ullman observes. Often, previous afflictions reoccur and then resolve as the remedy works through layers of healing, clearing the body of the residues of old illnesses. The rash soon disappeared.

In Sally's case, she needed six doses of the *Argentum nitricum* over the next three years, during which time she continued to improve. She is now a mother and doing "extremely well."

Homeopathic Nosodes: Anxiety and Vaccinations

In homeopathic terms, as noted previously, anxiety, like other disorders, is an imbalance of the vital force. Homeopaths have discovered that vaccinations are one of the environmental factors that can disturb an individual's vital force and produce a range of symptoms. Removing the adverse effects of vaccines in the body is the purview of a branch of homeopathy known as isopathy, which employs special remedies called nosodes.

Nosodes are homeopathic preparations of a pathogen. Many homeopaths include the use of nosodes under the rubric of homeopathy, but others prefer the term isopathy as a more accurate reflection of the practice. *Iso* means "equal," whereas *homeo* means "like." Nosodes are actually derived from the causative agent of a disease, whereas remedies are derived from substances that produce symptoms in a healthy person similar to a certain disease condition.

For example, the measles nosode is a dilution of the measles virus, and the MMR nosode is a dilution of the MMR vaccine. A homeopathic remedy often used to alleviate a case of measles is *Apis mellifica*, a dilution of a substance derived from bees. *Apis* is indicated for a skin rash that resembles bee stings in appearance and effect, which measles often does. *Apis* may alleviate symptoms of measles infection, but it will not clear the measles vaccine from the body, which the nosode can do. This homeopathic application is a single remedy to treat a transitory condition (measles), which is distinct from constitutional homeopathic treatment to rebalance the individual, as discussed in Dr. Reichenberg-Ullman's work.

It is important to note that a nosode, like other homeopathic remedies, does not actually contain any biochemical trace of the substance from which it is derived (in a nosode, a pathogen such as a virus), but is an energetic imprint of that substance. This is why nosodes do not produce the serious side effects associated with vaccines.

 For more about homeopathy and vaccines, see the author's *The Natural Medicine Guide to Autism* (Hampton Roads, 2002).

Nosodes: *Clearing Vaccine Reactions*

Nosodes can be highly effective in clearing adverse reactions to vaccines. The mechanism by which a nosode accomplishes this is not entirely understood, just as it is not fully understood how homeopathic remedies work to restore balance in the whole person. The effectiveness of nosodes is clearly demonstrated by clinical results, however, with a range of symptoms and conditions, including anxiety, disappearing after isopathic treatment.

In her practice, Carola M. Lage-Roy, a German homeopath (Heilpraktikerin Homoeopathie is the German medical credential she holds), has clearly seen the link between anxiety and vaccinations and has had extensive experience in using nosodes to reverse what she terms "vaccine damage."

Lage-Roy and her husband, Ravi Roy, have been practicing homeopathy as a team for more than 20 years, with offices in Murnau, Germany, and Encinitas, California. They direct a homeopathic research institute, teach around the world, and have written numerous books, including *Homoeopathic Guide: Vaccination Damage* and *The Homoeopathic Family Home-Care*.

Lage-Roy stresses the importance of reducing anxiety, beyond the obvious motivation of escaping the discomfort of it. "Anxiety is the cause of many problems in our lives," she observes. "The less anxiety we have, the more happiness and health we enjoy. So it is of fundamental importance to overcome this anxiety because it is the door that lets in diseases and all the other negative things that cause problems in your life. Fear is the door. We can see this very clearly in the world right now. The situation that is having a big impact on all of us is created by fear. The source behind war, terrorism, and the programs of vaccination to protect against germ warfare is fear."

As with other disorders, there is no one homeopathic remedy for fear (anxiety), but many remedies that work to resolve it. The appropriate remedy depends upon the individual's unique symptom picture and on the type of fears involved. For example, fear of being alone indicates a different remedy from fear of being with people.

The following case from Lage-Roy's patient files demonstrates the link between anxiety and vaccination, and the effectiveness of nosodes as treatment in cases where this link is a factor.

Joseph: *Panic and Polio*

When Joseph, 35, consulted Lage-Roy, he was already well-acquainted with homeopathy. He hoped that she could help with his severe anxiety and phobias, although a homeopath he had been seeing for years had been unable to do so. "His tremendous fear had not been influenced by homeopathy in any way," recalls Lage-Roy.

Joseph's anxiety was severely debilitating. His primary problem was claustrophobia. In his case, he believed that once he was in a room he wouldn't be able to get out. At these times, he felt like he was in prison. This fear applied to the cinema, the theatre, and the hair salon. He couldn't go get his hair cut because he was afraid he would not be able to get out of the salon.

Travel by train was equally problematic because a car on the train raised the same fear—that he would be unable to exit. The same thing happened when he tried to overcome his fears and visit friends in their homes, a tremendously stressful undertaking for him. The only way he could do this was by parking his car directly in front of his friend's house. Then when he became anxious inside the house, he could tell himself that the car was right out front and he could get away quickly.

The only place he felt safe was in his own house or in his car when he knew where he was going. He had a fear of getting lost, and walking anywhere was a problem for this reason. He was terrified that he would get lost and not be able to find his car, which meant again that he would be unable to escape from wherever he was. He was able to walk as long as he kept his car in sight, which naturally restricted his mobility.

Joseph suffered from xenophobia (fear of strangers) as well. Meeting new people brought on a panic attack. He was also afraid of using a toilet other than his own, which meant that he could not be away from home for long. This made travel, which was already a near impossibility given his other fears, entirely out of the question.

Joseph's symptoms began when he was 15 or 16, after he nearly fainted at school one day. From then on, school was highly stressful for him because the claustrophobia began at that point and he feared that he wouldn't be able to leave the classroom. He thought that he might have received a vaccine on the day that he fainted, but he wasn't completely sure. Three years later, at 18 or 19, he felt bad for some time after receiving his last polio vaccine, and his panic attacks got worse. This he was quite certain about, recalling it clearly.

When Lage-Roy heard this, she understood why the homeopathic treatment hadn't worked for Joseph. "It could not work because he was totally blocked by the vaccine," she explains. "Vaccines cause such a block in the whole system that the remedies can't work." There are other blocks that prevent remedies from working, but in this case, vaccines were the issue.

To remove the block and the adverse effects of the vaccines, she gave Joseph the polio nosode, a single dose at a 200D potency (the "D" stands for decimal; this is the same as a 200X potency).

Ten days later, Joseph reported in a letter to Lage-Roy, "The trend seems to be positive. There were some key situations in which I would have had a panic attack before taking the polio nosode." He gave the example of a friend's birthday party. Before, going to such an event would have filled him with panic, triggering all his major fears: leaving his house, being in a room he was afraid he wouldn't get out of, and meeting new people.

Joseph not only went to the party, but he drank some wine, which resulted in him feeling that he shouldn't drive. He was usually careful not to get himself into such situations. In the past, if this had happened, it would have brought on an extreme panic attack. He ended up sleeping overnight in his car, something he could never have done before, and everything was fine. Joseph thought that he probably drank the wine on purpose so he wouldn't be able to leave and would then have a chance to see his progress.

He also reported that since taking the remedy he didn't need the water in his morning shower to be as hot as before. This is significant, says Lage-Roy, because it signals an improvement in his life force, which had been depleted by the vaccines. "He was disconnected from the stream of vital energy, so he felt cold and needed a very hot shower to be revitalized in the morning."

Note that all of these improvements resulted from a single dose of the nosode.

Five days later, Joseph reported that he could now state that the action of the polio nosode was definitely positive. He could drive farther now without experiencing the panic that used to overtake him if he went too far. For the first time in his life, he was actually enjoying driving. He drove to the next town to meet a friend so they could walk their dogs together. This was another first for him.

Before taking the nosode, he had always needed an escape route to get away from any person he was with (he felt safest when he was alone). Without an escape route, he would be intensely uncomfortable. Joseph reported that he didn't feel that way anymore. He also expressed enthusiasm about what the future held. "I'm really curious and excited to see what will happen next with me."

A week later Joseph reported that his ongoing problem with flatulence and frequent stools, especially when he was experiencing stress, had disappeared. Within the month, he went to see a play for the first time in years. This development was especially significant as theatre etiquette requires that the audience remain in their seats during the play. Joseph was able to do so.

Two months after the initial dose of the polio nosode, Lage-Roy gave Joseph a second dose because he reported that the fear had returned a little. Immediately after taking this dose, he went through a healing crisis, during which the fear worsened briefly. (The healing crisis is a period during which symptoms temporarily worsen before finally breaking up; it is the turning point in healing, recognized by a range of natural medicine modalities.) Joseph felt fine after that and continued to improve from then on, with no relapses.

In summing up his progress, Joseph told Lage-Roy that his life had changed completely since taking the polio nosode. With his claustrophobia almost gone, he was living freely for the first time since his symptoms had appeared in his teens; he could travel, meet new people, go to the cinema and theatre. Two years later, he was still free from panic attacks.

In Joseph's case, all that was required to relieve his crippling anxiety were two doses of the polio nosode. "His was a clear case of vaccine damage," says Lage-Roy, adding that Joseph's former homeopath hadn't considered vaccines as a factor. "This was before many people were aware of the adverse effects of vaccines."

Lage-Roy notes that Joseph presented the classic picture of someone needing the polio nosode. Claustrophobia, panic attacks, and a deep impact on the bowel system, as evidenced by his flatulence and frequent stools, are all characteristic.

Treatment of vaccine-related anxiety is not always as simple as it was in Joseph's case. Lage-Roy recalls a 20-year-old man who nearly died after receiving a polio vaccine. He lost consciousness and collapsed. His legs were paralyzed after that. Like Joseph, he became afraid to leave his house. Interestingly, the young man's mother had the same fear. She too had suffered a strong reaction to, and become very ill after, a childhood polio vaccination. Of her inability to leave the house, she said that she felt as though there were a rubber band running between her belly button and the house. When she tried to leave, the band pulled her back.

As this man's mother was also a "vaccine victim," says Lage-Roy, "his genetic code was already influenced through this polio vaccine when he was born. So when he got the vaccine, it was much worse and he nearly died." Again, this young man had been treated by another homeopath, but the vaccine issue had not been addressed. He came to Lage-Roy and her husband after reading one of their books on vaccine damage. Homeopathic treatment restored the young man to health, but he needed numerous remedies, and it took longer than it had in Joseph's case.

Vaccines and Fear

Regarding the connection between vaccines and anxiety, Lage-Roy makes several astute observations. "Every vaccine causes a small inflammation in the brain," she says. "That is the desired effect because there has to be some reaction in the body that prompts the production of antibodies against the virus," which is the source of subsequent immunity according to the vaccine theory. Aside from the physical effects on the nervous system of such an inflammation, the brain is not equipped to deal with the reaction because it does not fit into the natural model of disease.

"By nature, disease is a learning process," says Lage-Roy. "It doesn't happen just by chance that you get sick. It's always the result of your lifestyle. It's always that you have to learn something through the disease." On the most simplistic level, the lesson you need to learn might be that you have a tendency to overextend yourself, to work and play too hard, and illness provides an opportunity for you to learn that you need to slow down.

Through vaccines, however, you are attacked by the disease, but this disease did not arise naturally as a life lesson for you because it was injected into you rather than contracted in the course of life. In addition, there is no learning process in nature that puts you through five diseases at the same time, as immunizations containing multiple vaccines do.

Further, there are several direct connections between fear and vaccines, says Lage-Roy. "All the vaccines are connected with anxiety because the driving force to get the vaccine *is* anxiety because you are afraid of getting the disease, or your parents or your school are afraid of you getting the disease."

Vaccines are also derived from substances foreign to the

human body: the chemical additives, the disease organisms, and in some cases the culture in which the organisms are grown. For instance, a widely used version (IPOL) of the Salk (injected) polio vaccine is grown in a culture of monkey kidney cells, extracted from laboratory animals. The latter adds the monkey's fear at being kept in a cage in a sterile environment and subjected to scientific procedures to the human fear associated with vaccines, explains Lage-Roy. In summary, the energy imprint of all the fear is in the vaccine.

In further corroboration of the fear-vaccine connection, Lage-Roy reports that she sees in her practice a big difference between children who have never been vaccinated and those who have. It's quite obvious, she says. Parents who had their first child vaccinated before they knew of the dangers and then declined to have a second child vaccinated have commented to her on the difference they see between the two, and their observations concur with hers. "Children who have not been vaccinated are more free, have higher self-esteem, are sick less often, and have much less fear and anxiety," says Lage-Roy.

Parents need to know that there are safe alternatives to immunizations. Homeopathic nosodes can be used instead of vaccinations and also to clear vaccine reactions from the body if conventional immunizations have been used. If a child does happen to contract measles, mumps, chicken pox, or other ailment, homeopathic remedies can ease the severity of the illness and shorten its duration. There are also safer ways to vaccinate your child if you decide to go the conventional route. Safer vaccination policies include vaccinating later, giving vaccines separately instead of in combination, allowing two months between vaccines, and monitoring vaccine reactions (another vaccine should not be administered until it is clear there are no complications).[162]

For adults who suspect that vaccine reactions might be a component in their or their child's anxiety disorder, consulting a homeopath who is versed in the use of nosodes to clear vaccine reactions may be beneficial.

6 Energy Medicine III: Flower Essence Therapy

Like homeopathy, flower essence therapy works on an energetic level to restore the equilibrium of the body, mind, and spirit. The particular specialty of flower essences is the realm of emotions and attitudes, which exert a powerful influence on health and ill health. As Edward Bach, an English physician and homeopath and the father of flower essence therapy, stated it, "Behind all disease lie our fears, our anxieties, our greed, our likes and dislikes."[163] By addressing underlying psychospiritual issues and promoting energetic shifts in the mind and emotions, flower essences promote a return to health on all levels.

Put simply, flower essences are "catalysts to mind-body wellness," explains Patricia Kaminski, co-director of the Flower Essence Society in Nevada City, California, and a renowned innovator in the field of flower essence therapy for more than 20 years (see "What Is Flower Essence Therapy?"). Or you could say they act as a bridge between the realms of the physical and the spiritual, the body and the soul.[164]

As homeopath Carola Lage-Roy pointed out in the previous chapter, every illness, including anxiety, contains a lesson for the person afflicted. From the viewpoint of flower essence therapy, this lesson regards a psychospiritual issue that is not being dealt with or a psychospiritual need that is not being met, says Kaminski. These neglected areas of the individual create energy imbalances that over time can manifest in illness. By helping to bring psychospiritual issues and unmet needs to light, flower essences facilitate the resolution of these issues, rebalancing of the attendant energy disturbances, and restoration of health.

A purely biochemical model fails to address the emotional, psychological, and spiritual components of anxiety. Manipulating brain chemistry, as with anti-anxiety drugs, may mask the symptoms of anxiety, but it does nothing to correct the root causes of the anxiety. If brain chemistry is skewed, what caused that to happen? According to the flower essence model, the biochemical imbalances found in anxiety are caused by the distress of the spirit, or soul, says Kaminski. Thus, a purely biochemical approach will not cure anxiety because it does not deal with the source—the soul's crisis.

The embrace of the biochemical model in medicine reflects our cultural bias for physical development over psychospiritual development, she observes. For example, exercising the body to develop its strength or undergoing physical therapy to redevelop strength after a stroke or an injury are standard and widespread practices. But a similar emphasis on psychospiritual development in "mental disorders" is lacking. Instead, medical intervention seeks to remove the symptoms as quickly as possible. "We intervene earlier and earlier when someone is in emotional pain and distress," states Kaminski. "We use biochemical therapies to 'fix' the problem at its current level of symptom manifestation, rather than encouraging further psychological development."

This is where flower essences can be a valuable tool. "The approach of flower essence therapy is to recognize the dignity of the human soul and to recognize the capacity of the human soul to change and become stronger," she elaborates. "The soul isn't connected to the aging of the body, so even if you're 70 years old, you can still be developing from the point of view of the soul. What we want to look at when somebody is facing a crisis, when they present with anxiety, with depression, with an addiction, is: what is it that the soul is really facing? . . . There's enormous capacity in the human spirit and the human soul to acquire skills for transforming what is a problem into a gift, if the therapy goes deep enough."

What Is Flower Essence Therapy?

The use of flower essences is often dismissed in the United States, even by some alternative medicine practitioners, as a "lightweight" therapy that may be pleasing but has little therapeutic value. One reason for the misconception may be the general lack of understanding in this country about energy medicine, which is widely accepted in Europe. As the promising results of scientific investigation into flower essence therapy and other forms of energy medicine are mounting and an increasing number of alternative medicine physicians and other health care professionals are routinely employing these modalities, the misconceptions are gradually being dispelled. More people are discovering the truth about flower essence therapy, which is that it has the capability to stimulate profound change on a deep level, Kaminski states.

To clarify another common misunderstanding, essential oils (aromatherapy) and flower essences are two different kinds of medicine. While essential oils contain the biochemical components of the plants from which they are extracted, flower essences are closer to homeopathic remedies in nature, in that they are energetic imprints of their source. Another way of saying this is that a flower essence contains the life force of the flower.

A flower essence is made by sun-infusing the blossoms of a particular plant, bush, or tree in water. (This is a simplistic summary of the process, which involves timing the picking of the flowers according to life-cycle, environmental, and other factors.) The liquid is then diluted and potentized in a method similar to the preparation of homeopathic remedies, and preserved with brandy (or a nonalcoholic substance, if need be). The result is a highly diluted, potentized substance that embodies the energetic patterns of the flower from which it is made. This means that the therapeutic effects of flower essences are vibrational or energetic.[165]

Despite Einstein and solid science demonstrating that matter is energy, the fact that you can contain energy in a liquid and influence human energy fields to help resolve ailments is not widely known. Yet, that is precisely what flower essence liquids do. When you take flower essences, the energy they contain affects your energy field, which in turn has an impact on your physical, mental, emotional, and spiritual condition, as these aspects are all energy based.

In the 1930s, Dr. Edward Bach developed 38 different flower essences to address 38 different emotional-soul or psychological types. As an example of the "profile" associated with a remedy, the flower essence Willow is indicated for someone who, when out of balance, feels resentful, bitter, and envious of others and adopts a "poor me" victim stance. Dr. Bach's remedies are still available today—the Bach Flower Remedies seen in health food stores everywhere.

The Flower Essence Society (FES) in Nevada City, California, headed by Kaminski and her husband, Richard Katz, has expanded on the work of Dr. Bach and significantly furthered the field of flower essences. Founded in 1979 by Katz, FES is a pioneer in flower essence research, compiling and analyzing case study data from tens of thousands of practitioners around the world and conducting longitudinal studies as well as botanical field studies.

FES also funds double-blind placebo trials with specific flower essences. In two such studies, clinical and research psychologist Jeffrey Cram, Ph.D., director of the Sierra Health Institute in Nevada City, looked at the efficacy of specific flower essence formulas in alleviating stress. Physiological measures showed significantly reduced reactivity in subjects who received the flower essences versus those given a placebo.[166]

Currently under way is a major study on the application of flower essences in depression.[167]

In addition to the society's involvement in research, Kaminski and Katz expanded on Bach's remedies, developing a line of more than 100 flower essences derived from North American plants. They developed the line (the FES brand, also found in many health food stores) to expand the emotional repertoire of flower essences; to provide North Americans with essences derived from indigenous plants, which might better resonate with their healing issues; and to address the more complicated emotional and psychological makeup of people today.

 There are many flower essence practitioners. The Flower Essence Society operates a Practitioner Referral Network, with a listing of about 3,000 flower essence therapists in the U.S. and Canada alone; contact Flower Essence Society, P.O. Box 459, Nevada City, CA 95959; tel: 530-265-9163 or 800-736-9222; website: www.flowersociety.org.

The Soul Message in Anxiety

While every person is different and the causes of anxiety are many, Patricia Kaminski has observed in her practice a common theme, or soul message, if you will. "The underlying soul predicament with anxiety is fear, and underlying that fear is a lack in the ability to meet the world, to take on the world. The virtue that is lacking is courage."

The definition of courage that for her best describes the relationship of fear and courage in flower essence therapy comes from Rudolph Giuliani, the former mayor of New York City, who said during the crisis after the 9/11 attacks, "Courage is realizing you're afraid and still acting." In flower essence terms, the therapy does not get rid of the fear, but helps people to find the courage to move forward in their lives even though they are afraid.

This is in sharp contrast to the pharmaceutical approach, which tranquilizes the system in order to suppress the fear. "Somehow we believe that if we could just take something, then we wouldn't have fear," says Kaminski. "But there is always going to be fear, particularly in the culture we live in now, with bioterrorism, etc. We're not going to get rid of fear. But what is within the capacity of the human soul to do is to meet the fear and act anyway."

In contrast with depression, which is a kind of shutting down of the body—a lethargic condition—anxiety is a speeded-up con-

Flower Essences for Anxiety

While every person is different and flower essence therapy must be tailored to the individual, the following are flower essences commonly indicated in cases of anxiety:

- Aspen: anxiety that is often psychic in origin, or unexplained foreboding and dread

- Five-Flower Formula (Bach's Rescue Remedy): emergency stress situations; to alleviate acute anxiety when specific remedy needed is unclear

- Garlic: chronic worry and anxiety; stage fright

- Golden Yarrow: performance anxiety, especially felt in the solar plexus (upper abdominal region)

- Larch: fear of failure

- Mimulus: fear of known things

- Mustard: free-floating anxiety, accompanied by symptoms of manic-depression

Sources: Patricia Kaminski and Richard Katz, Flower Essence Repertory, *Nevada City, CA: Flower Essence Society, 1996. "The Original Bach Flower Essences," booklet published by Nelson Bach USA, Ltd., Philadelphia, PA, 1995.*

dition, with the body going into overdrive, as typified by the heart palpitations, rapid pulse, and sweating, she explains. While in depression the emotional challenge is to contact buried feelings; in anxiety the challenge is to gain emotional objectivity and not allow certain emotions to take over.

People with anxiety disorders "need to step back from a kind of hyper-emotional reaction to life," Kaminski states. "They need calming, but not as in shutting the doors and not going out into life. What they need to develop is courage to meet life, and to trust life on its own terms." Flower essences can help anxious people *meet* life instead of shrinking from it.

From the flower essence perspective, it is important to consider any disorder as a spectrum within the possibilities of a human being, says Kaminski. This means that, while some people are on the extreme end of the anxiety spectrum, suffering from severe phobias or obsessive-compulsive disorder, for example, we all carry those conditions within us, and given the right circumstances we could develop them. "I've known people in prison who started to develop certain aspects of those disorders because of the enormous stress and fear of that experience. We all could be pressed into these corners of the human psyche."

Given the level of fear in our society today, it is important for us to find healing approaches that help us deal with fear. Flower essence therapy is one of these.

Kaminski cautions against approaching flower essence therapy in a mode similar to drug treatment, merely substituting a natural product for the chemical, in the hopes that the medicine will get rid of the fear more safely. Certainly, a natural approach is preferable where possible, but to regard any substance as the "magic bullet" that will fix a disorder is to misunderstand the true nature of healing. Yes, there are flower essences that work quickly to calm a person in an emergency situation, notably Rescue Remedy (also known as Five-Flower Remedy). "But an emergency intervention formula will not work over the long haul with something like an anxiety disorder," notes Kaminski.

Truly dealing with anxiety and other "mental" disorders through flower essence therapy involves working in layers, and it is a process, not a quick fix, says Kaminski. "It's a whole developmental process for the soul. The developmental process involves steps—metamorphoses that have to happen. We have to work in

> **Truly dealing with anxiety and other "mental" disorders through flower essence therapy involves working in layers, and it is a process, not a quick fix, says Kaminski. "It's a whole developmental process for the soul. The developmental process involves steps—metamorphoses that have to happen."**

a way to bring the consciousness up in the person. Whereas in typical medicine, we mask the consciousness, what we do with flower essences is try to stimulate the consciousness to see these pictures, these parts of the soul."

The following case history is based on information provided by the "patient" herself, Kendra Barnett of Nevada City, California. Although she was not treated by Kaminski, she became her student. Kendra was so impressed by how flower essences were able to release her from severe anxiety and depression that she went on to complete the Flower Essence Society's practitioner training program so she could help others discover the healing power of this therapy. Her story offers the unique perspective of the healed and the healer.

Kendra: Stopped by Fear

At 16, Kendra was put on an antidepressant due to her severe anxiety and depression. She had frequent panic attacks when she was at school, at work, or in another public place. At these times, she was filled with fear, her heart raced, she felt like she couldn't breathe, and she wanted to get home where no one could see her. Her fear was of people looking at her and of them seeing her do something wrong. These symptoms are characteristic of social anxiety disorder.

"When I was out in public, I felt very vulnerable and I would have anxiety attacks," she says. "Then I would go home, feel terrible about being like that, and get really depressed. That was my cycle."

Kendra avoided the panic attacks by staying home, so consequently missed a lot of school. "I hung out by myself because I was in a dark space inside. I felt empty and stuck," she recalls. "I wasn't being creative. I couldn't find any inner motivation. I was just a stuck teenager."

On a scale of one to ten, with ten being most severe, Kendra rated her condition as at the top of the scale. She would be better at some times than others, but her panic attacks were "tens," she recalls. There didn't seem to be an external reason for her state, as her childhood had been a happy one and she had a "wonderful family."

The antidepressant didn't offer Kendra much relief. Although it lessened the depression a little, she still felt empty inside and still had the panic attacks. The drug also didn't do anything for her feeling of being stuck. "It wasn't moving me forward in my life," she says. "I was frustrated. I knew there was more for me in my life, but I didn't have any skills or tools to help me move forward."

Kendra had a job in a store that sold flower essences. She hadn't heard about them before that. Over time, she learned that flower essences were especially good in the emotional arena. That prompted her to go to her doctor and ask about the possibility of taking flower essences. The doctor advised her not to go off the drug. "The doctor said they wouldn't work and that I would probably never come off antidepressants." Not knowing any better, Kendra discarded the idea of flower essences.

Two years after she had begun taking the antidepressant, her condition was much the same. One day at work, Kendra's boss witnessed one of her panic attacks. She could see Kendra's tremendous anxiety, and there was nothing happening around her to prompt it, so it was clear that it arose from within. "I felt so horrible that she was witnessing it," recalls Kendra, "but she grabbed a flower essence bottle and said, 'Here, take this.' It was Mimulus, which is for fear of known things. As soon as I held the Mimulus in my hand, it was like a big sigh came out of my heart. I actually physically sighed."

Just from holding the bottle, Kendra felt a shift in her. "I haven't had a panic attack since that day, and I haven't taken medication since then either." From that moment, Kendra stopped taking the antidepressant and began taking the standard flower essence dose of four drops four times a day. (Note that it is not recommended to discontinue psychiatric medications without medical supervision. A gradual tapering off of the dosage is the method generally advised in order to avoid ill effects. Kendra was fortunate in that she had no adverse reactions to her abrupt discontinuation.)

"I stopped taking the drug immediately after I discovered the Mimulus because the flower essence gave me an inner light, inside my heart. The Mimulus flower is yellow, like the sun. Also, my anxiety was centered in my solar plexus (stomach), and the color of that chakra is yellow. The Mimulus helped my stomach not to be churning with anxiety." She also noticed that the flower essence began to fill her with self-worth, and the feeling of emptiness subsided. The flower essence didn't get rid of her fear, but gave her the message that the emotions she was feeling were fine and that it was possible to look at them in different ways.

"I started moving forward, one step at a time. That was what I had needed—a catalyst." She began to go out in the world more, started studying aromatherapy and, later, flower essences. Meanwhile, Kendra's boss at the store taught her more about flower essences, and she began to take others as she felt she needed them.

The ones that were particularly helpful, in addition to Mimulus, were Crab Apple and Walnut. "Crab Apple helps to cleanse you of feeling unclean and impure. That was important for me, too. The emptiness inside of me made me feel gunky. There wasn't a lot of light. The Crab Apple helped me to cleanse and move forward. Walnut is also for moving forward with courage."

Kendra, now 25, regards Mimulus as an ongoing healing and still takes it today, although not at the original dosage. "I'm continually taking flower essences," she says. "I take a different blend every month. I still get anxious, but nothing like before. I get healthy anxiety. Sometimes I feel a little bit vulnerable when I'm putting myself out there in the world or I notice that I'm falling back into my old pattern, and I just put some Mimulus back into my blend. It's like a best friend."

She views Mimulus as the archetypal essence for this time in her life. "The Mimulus gives me the courage to go on with my life and not worry about the little things, like people looking at me or seeing me do something wrong. It was those little anxieties that became unhealthy and interfered with my functioning. The Mimulus gives me the courage to do what I have to do and to be myself."

In looking back at her anxiety and depression, she thinks that they may have been an outgrowth of getting stuck in the transition from childhood to adulthood. "All teenagers go through some sort of change. They need to find where they need to go, and they need to have positive inspiration. I got stuck in that transition. I had no insight."

Kendra found it difficult to talk to anyone about her depression and panic attacks and, like many young people, felt that nobody understood her. After the antidepressant didn't work, she didn't think there was anything that could help her. "I wanted to get better, I wanted to enjoy my life, but I didn't have the tools."

Fortunately, Kendra found a tool that worked to get her moving again. Flower essences helped summon qualities in her that she didn't know how to bring out on her own. "The pharmaceutical drugs didn't fill me up inside with the love and wonder and beauty of life," she says, which is what she needed and what the flower essences did for her. "I was empty inside. I needed to come from a whole place in myself before I could go out into the world."

Kendra echoes Kaminski's point that true healing is not a quick fix. "To get to your core issues is a big journey that not everyone wants to take. I was willing to take responsibility for everything inside of me, and I think that's one reason the flower essences helped me. I feel like I got to the core, and every day now I'm really light. Now the rest of my life is just unfolding, and it's a wonderful journey."

Kendra reports that at this point she has tried almost all of the Bach and FES remedies and has found them all helpful. They bring forth the rainbow of human qualities that are already there, but need help in coming out into the world, she says.

Flower essences are a direct path not only to connection with all aspects of being human, but also to connection with the natural world. "We're so concerned right now with the material world. We need to connect more with nature. When we do, we connect with ourselves." Kendra observes that the sense of beauty and wonder you get from walking through a forest or being in your garden is how she feels when she takes the flower essences. Since you can't always be in your garden or walking in a forest, flower essences are a way to keep that sense of connection, beauty, and wonder in your everyday life, she notes, which can go a long way toward dissolving anxiety.

The Medication of Souls

"It's not easy working with anxiety and depression in our culture, because of the tremendous emphasis on medication,"

Kaminski states. "The longer somebody has been on psychiatric drugs, the more challenges we have. The sooner we can get to somebody, if they have been on the drugs for a short time, the more successful we're going to be. That's actually true of both flower essences and homeopathy."

It's not that people who have been on pharmaceuticals for a long time can't be helped by flower essences. It just makes the case more complex, she says. The flower essence practitioner has to work then with the chemical situation that has been set up in the body as well as with the emotional layers.

Kaminski cautions that this is not to say that people should simply throw away their prescription drugs. Stopping needs to be done under the supervision of a qualified physician, and obviously if someone is suicidal or psychotic, the drugs may be saving their life.

Like Dr. Reichenberg-Ullman, Kaminski has a vision of another way that people can be helped in times of crisis. She would like to see doctors put patients whose "mental" disorders are not life-threatening on flower essences *first*. "That's what's happening in Cuba," she states. "The flower essences have become part of the medical model there. They've seen the results." The Cuban Ministry of Public Health recognizes flower essence therapy as a valid medical modality and has sponsored practitioner training in its use in ten of the country's 15 provinces.[168]

Kaminski adds: "What I would like to see is a revolution in the health-care industry, that at the early stages of intervention, when somebody needs emotional help, we provide, in addition to counseling, therapeutic modalities that are much safer and much more holistic. If those don't work, then we can consider stronger chemical options."

Again, with somebody who's suicidal or psychotic, immediate brain intervention in the form of medication may be necessary. "If your hand is in the fire, you can't go right to giving a remedy for healing the hand," says Kaminski. "The first thing you have to do is get the hand out of the fire." It's important to remember, however, that a tranquilizer or an antidepressant is never a cure, she cautions. Rather, it only temporarily changes behavior and enables the brain to function differently.

Unfortunately, those facts seem to have been forgotten. Kaminski points to an alarming trend in the use of pharmaceuticals. "It's just unconscionable to me how many people are being put on psychiatric drugs at the drop of a hat." Statistics on the huge increase in the prescription of such drugs over the past two decades demonstrate what Kaminski calls "the normalization of psychiatry."

In other words, she says, "more and more and more of the population is being medicated. If somebody comes in suffering from lethargy, panic, anxiety, or PTSD [posttraumatic stress disorder], we right away medicate them. Children are being medicated. The elderly are being medicated. Prisoners are being medicated." What medication does is rob individuals of the capacity to deal with their soul and the messages it has to communicate, she says. "Whether it's conscious or unconscious, we're actually developing a model that is robbing people of their developmental capacity. There is a trend, both in psychiatry and in medicine, to medicate away problems."

The use of psychiatric drugs is behavior modification to help people adjust to their lives the way they are, according to Kaminski. "It isn't a transformative model of a human being. It's a behavioral adaptive model." She sees the results of this in people who come to her who have been on psychiatric drugs for a while—there is no movement in their lives.

The psychiatric drug model also seems to be promoting the idea that "we're supposed to somehow have the smiley face all the time," she observes. "The truth of the matter is, life hurts. There are failures and disappointments."

Kaminski envisions the development of a different model of human potential, one that doesn't only seek to fix, but asks why the breakdown happened. "What's standing in the way of that person being able to move on, to be a more loving and more productive person in human society? That for me is the goal of flower essence therapy—to wake people up, even if it's painful. When we open our heart to take risks, then our lives are more healthy, they're more whole."

7 Cellular Memory and Structural Issues: Soma Therapies

Cellular memory is another aspect of the emotional component of anxiety, according to Zannah Steiner, C.M.P., R.M.T., founder and clinic director of Soma Therapy Centre in Vancouver, British Columbia. The body remembers all the traumas an individual has experienced, whether physical injury or emotional upset, because the attendant emotions are stored in the body's tissues, she explains. This is what is known as cellular memory. While psychotherapy can help uncover many of the issues involved in the emotional component of anxiety, it may not effect the release of cellular memories underlying the anxiety, and so resolution is not achieved.

In Steiner's experience, anxiety also typically involves structural factors, meaning a misalignment in the body from birth or injury. While addressing the structural aspect can produce significant changes in anxiety, unless the emotional components are addressed as well, the structural balance may be thrown off again, "because we are body, mind, and spirit," she states. Correcting only one will not produce long-lasting benefits.

Steiner's expertise in the mind-body relationship stems not only from 20 years as a registered massage therapist, but also a decade of study with osteopathic physician John Upledger, the originator of CranioSacral Therapy and SomatoEmotional Release (see "Soma Therapies"). Through this work, she has gained a deep understanding of the relationship between emotional states and the body's structure. She founded Soma Therapy Centre to bring under one roof a variety of soma therapies that she has found work well together to fully restore balance in the mind and body. Through these therapies, stored trauma can be released and structural misalignment corrected.

Let's look at the structural issues that can be involved in anxiety and then return to the emotional aspect and the concept of cellular memory.

The Structure of Anxiety

The body's structure in this case refers mainly to the bones at either pole of the craniosacral system: the sacrum (base of the spine) and the cranium (the skull). If these bones are out of alignment, the function of the craniosacral system can be thrown off. Structural distortion in the body produces compression. Compression or compaction is constriction due to pressure exerted on a body part or system. If the distortion is in the bones of the skull, for example, the result can be compression or a pressing on the brain and cranial nerves.

Such distortion and compression affect the flow of the fluid that bathes the brain and spinal cord, called cerebrospinal fluid (CSF). Normally, CSF flows up and down the spine in a kind of rhythmic tide. When CSF is not flowing properly, it has a profound impact on the brain, nervous system, and entire body. (See "Soma Therapies" for a more detailed explanation of the craniosacral system.) Anxiety is one of many conditions that can result from structural misalignment and the attendant disturbed CSF flow.

Further, there is a vicious cycle, called the "viscerosomatic reflex," that occurs in the body during anxiety or panic, says Steiner. Constriction in the organs (viscera)—the tight feeling in the lungs, heart, and stomach that typically attends anxious feelings—sends messages to the nervous system, which "engages the person emotionally in a relentness kind of pain-tension cycle. The heightened experience of both the nervous system and the person's response to it can easily compound both the visceral and the emotional components of the situation, escalating it and accelerating it to a disproportionate scale."

Through soma therapies, the vicious cycle of the viscerosomatic reflex can be interrupted, and structural and functional factors corrected.

The "Terrible Triad"

While every individual is unique and there is no anxiety template, a common structural component involved in both anxiety and depression is what Dr. Upledger termed "the terrible triad."

The terrible triad means a state of compression between the sacrum (base of the spine), the sphenoid (a bone that, in part, forms the orbits of the eyes), and the occiput (the occipital bone, or back of the skull). In other words, these bone structures produce constriction on the brain and dural membranes (the membranes covering the brain and spinal cord) and restrict the flow of CSF.

It is important to note at this point that the bones of the skull are not fixed, as many people believe. The skull "breathes" with the ebbing and flowing of the cerebrospinal fluid. Problems result when the bones become immobile due to misalignment, as is the case in the terrible triad, and the CSF "breathing" is impaired.

In the skull, the temporal bones (the bones that the ears sit in) come together with the sphenoid and the occipital bones at flexible joints. The flexibility of these articulations between the skull bones is impeded when the temporal bones are in an asynchronous condition. This means they are moving in opposition to each other with the ebb and flow of CSF, instead of together as they are meant to do. Asynchrony of the temporal bones sets the stage for the terrible triad.

When the temporal bones are not moving synchronously, this restricts the normal movement of the bones of the head and the dural membranes. This, in turn, transmits tension all the way down the spinal cord to the sacrum, thereby reducing expansion and retraction and subsequently production and distribution of cerebrospinal fluid. The result is decreased mobility of the body in general and compromise of the immune and other systems, as

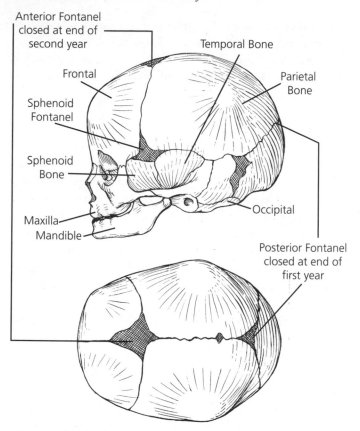

Fontanels of Infant's Skull and the Main Bones of Skull
The sphenoid, occipital, and temporal bones of the
skull are involved in the "terrible triad."

CSF is vital to their operation. Thus, rigidity and compression in the skull can have far-reaching neurological, functional, mental, and behavioral effects.

The terrible triad can result from birth trauma or later physical trauma such as a car accident, chronic injury, or systemic infection. Fortunately, CranioSacral Therapy can release the compression in the craniosacral system and break up the terrible triad.

Steiner and other CST practitioners have found that this pattern is often present in anxiety disorders, particularly PTSD (posttraumatic stress disorder). One study of Vietnam veterans who suffered from PTSD found that significant improvement in their symptoms occurred following release of the components forming the terrible triad.[169]

Cellular Memory

The body's storage of the emotions felt during traumatic events is an often overlooked source of anxiety. Treatment rarely addresses this cellular memory, and so it lingers in the body and fuels anxiety

A trauma results in the formation of what Dr. Upledger termed "energy cysts" as the body walls off the trauma to store it locally rather than allowing it to become systemic. Just as the body creates inflammation around the puncture site after you step on a nail, it forms an energy cyst in the body to contain the residues of strong emotions such as fear, anger, or resentment that remain in the body after a traumatic emotional event.

> **The body's storage of the emotions felt during traumatic events is an often overlooked source of anxiety. Treatment rarely addresses this cellular memory, and so it lingers in the body and fuels anxiety.**

For example, if as a child your mother looked at you with eyes like daggers, your body may have experienced it like a stab to the heart. The body then walled off the energetic residues in that area, creating an energy cyst in your chest. Or the residues could be stored in muscles or organs somewhere else in the body. These energy cysts restrict the body's free flow of energy and movement, may produce discomfort, and become a localized source of dysfunction.[170]

Emotional residues can be stored in energy cysts anywhere in the body, including in organs. "The cellular memory in that energy cyst can be visual, kinesthetic [related to movement], auditory, or all of the above," Steiner explains. As the emotions are released from the energy cysts during SomatoEmotional Release (see "Soma Therapies"), patients reexperience the emotions and may remember the event involved. They may even assume the position they were in when the injury or trauma occurred.

As with all of the therapies used at Soma Therapy Centre, in SomatoEmotional Release the therapists take their cue from the patient's body. "We follow the body," explains Steiner. "If you were to feel in your own body the position that your body is inclined to go into, that would be the position that we would follow. Ultimately, it would take us to the injury that caused the position, so at the depths of that movement pattern is the original injury. You might have a memory of it. You might say, 'Oh, this is the fall from the tricycle at age three.'" Release can take place, however, even without the cognitive recall of the memory.

Soma Therapies

The following techniques are the primary therapies used by Zannah Steiner and her colleagues at Soma Therapy Centre to address the structural, functional, and emotional components of anxiety and other disorders:

CranioSacral Therapy (CST): This technique was developed by John Upledger, D.O., who defined CST as a "hands-on method of evaluating and enhancing the functioning of a physiological body system called the craniosacral system—comprised of the dural membranes and cerebrospinal fluid (CSF) that surround and protect the brain and spinal cord."[171] The word "craniosacral" derives from the two poles of this system: the sacrum (base of the spine) and the cranium (the skull).

The skull is composed of interlocking bones that are far more mobile than most people think. Accident, injury, and the birth process can cause misalignment of the bone plates, resulting in what is termed cranial distortion. This distortion can in turn exert pressure on the brain (compression), impede the proper flow of CSF, and compromise the function of the nervous system.

The craniosacral system, which drives the flow of cerebrospinal fluid, operates as a semi-closed hydraulic pumping mechanism. "That pumping mechanism is responsible for ensuring that all of the fluids of the body are flowing," says Steiner. "Cerebrospinal fluid is the body's most important fluid. It is the basic 'soup stock' of the body, containing the ingredients—proteins, enzymes, and electrolytes—that are the basis of all other fluid systems." When CSF flow is diminished, fewer nutrients and less oxygen are delivered, and all other fluid systems are compromised. Thus, less CSF means less of everything else.

Compression in the skull and the attendant impeded CSF flow can produce symptoms throughout the body, from the more obvious such as headaches and back pain to the less obvious such as breathing and digestive disorders.[172]

Examination using CST protocols (which include evaluation of the craniosacral system) determines the status of cerebrospinal fluid flow and nervous system function. By releasing restrictions in the craniosacral system through gentle manipulations, CST improves central nervous system function and has beneficial effects for many health conditons.

According to the Upledger Institute in Palm Beach Gardens, Florida, these include central nervous system disorders, emotional difficulties, posttraumatic stress disorder (PTSD), chronic fatigue, stress and tension-related problems, immune disorders, motor-coordination impairments, colic, autism, learning disabilities, fibromyalgia and other connective-tissue disorders, temporo-mandibular joint syndrome (TMJ), orthopedic problems, migraine headaches, and chronic neck and back pain.[173]

SomatoEmotional Release (SER): An offshoot of CST, SER is a hands-on technique developed around 1980 by Dr. Upledger and biophysicist Zvi Karni, Ph.D. SER works to aid the body in releasing the residual effects (energy cysts) of past traumas, which can be emotional; viral; bacterial; or physical, as from an injury or structural damage.

Through contacting the energy cysts via touch, the therapist works with the patient's body-mind to release the emotional content of the blockages, relying on the messages communicated by the craniosacral system as a guide.

While some patients engage with the therapist in what is termed in SER "reflective dialogue technique," talking about what they are feeling in the process, the experience need not be articulated. It is as effective on a preverbal or nonverbal level, which makes SER an excellent method for releasing the residues of past traumas in infants and children.

The release of energy cysts often produces immediate emotional and physical benefits. As SER helps restore the free flow of energy and movement in the body, the conditions that can be ameliorated by the therapy may be limitless. Among those that Zannah Steiner cites as responding well are mental disorders, neurological disorders, chronic pain, whiplash, and degenerative diseases.

Process Oriented Counseling: Also called Process Work, this is a therapeutic method developed by Jungian analyst Dr. Arnold Mindell. It approaches areas of an individual's life that he or she experiences as "problematic or painful" and seeks to discover without judgment the meaning of and potential for personal growth contained in those areas. Symptoms in the body are "traced to their origin, whether they are of a physical, mental, emotional, and/or spiritual nature," Zannah Steiner explains. Process Work can aid CranioSacral Therapy in effecting the release of emotional issues stored in the body.

Visceral Manipulation: This therapeutic technique for relieving restrictions and tensions in and around organs (viscera) was developed by French osteopath Jean-Pierre Barral in the early 1970s. "The basic philosophy of Visceral Manipulation is that an organ in good health has good movement," Zannah Steiner explains. When tissue becomes rigid or fixed, chronic irritation and dysfunction result. The function of surrounding tissue is also compromised as the tissue attempts to adapt to the change.

According to Dr. Barral, each organ in the body has its own biological rhythm, moving through five to eight cycles per minute. It actually moves subtly in a rotation around what Dr. Barral termed its own "embryogenic axis" or fulcrum, which is the orientation it had when the fetal organs were developing. Scar tissue from surgery or injury, chronic inflammation, or shortened fascia (fibrous connective tissue) can disturb the rhythm and suspension (rotation) of organs. Through specifically applied light manual force, Visceral Manipulation releases the tensions and restrictions, and restores the proper mobility and inherent rhythm of the organs. As poor flow of cerebrospinal fluid can interfere with organ function, CranioSacral Therapy is an important adjunct.

In addition to improved organ function, resulting benefits are better fluid circulation, relief of sphincter and muscle spasms, relief of chronic pain and tension, improved digestion and hormonal balance, and enhancement of localized and systemic immunity. "The organ system can be a storage facility of unexpressed emotion," says Steiner. "The organs are thought to contain the 'voice of the body.'" Thus, Visceral Manipulation can also release emotional holding. With the therapy, patients often experience a sense of well-being.[174]

 For information about CST, SER, and VM, contact the Upledger Institute/American CranioSacral Therapy Association, 11211 Prosperity Farms Rd., Ste. D-325, Palm Beach Gardens, FL 33410; tel: 561-622-4334; website: www.upledger.com. For CST, see the Canadian College of Osteopathy, Toronto, Ontario; website: www.osteopathy-canada.ca. For Process Oriented Counseling, see the website of Dr. Arnold Mindell (www.aamindell.net), or contact Process Work Center of Portland, 2049 NW Hoyt St., Ste. 1, Portland, OR 97209; tel: 503-223-8188; website: www.processwork.org.

The Soma Approach

It's important to note that Steiner, like many natural medicine practitioners, does not rely on conventional diagnostic labels such as panic disorder to guide her treatment approach. "We do an assessment of each patient without knowing anything about their history," says Steiner. Treatment is then designed according to those findings, rather than being dictated by a label, symptom, or condition. An anxiety disorder may be the indication for treatment, but there may be many other things happening in an individual that are causing it. Approaching a patient in this way allows for genuine treatment of that person at a deep level.

In addition, patients are viewed with new eyes at each visit, even if the visits are on consecutive days. This allows for adjustment in approach to changes that may have occurred as the result of the previous treatment or other factors. "We treat each patient as a completely new patient each time they come," says Steiner. "Otherwise, we'd be bringing an agenda or a bias into the treatment." This means that as patients move through layers of healing, the therapy moves with them.

The approach Steiner has found most effective is an intensive week of therapy (two weeks is optimum), which means being treated five hours a day for five days in succession, predominantly with CST, Visceral Manipulation, and SER, but other therapies are used as needed. This program "bombards people's nervous systems to the point that they move through their issues in a week or two weeks," says Steiner.

A "good percentage" of the Centre's patients (and likely a good percentage of the population at large as well) have suffered some form of abuse—whether physical, sexual, surgical, emotional, or spiritual abuse—and this intensive approach enables people to release their cellular memories of the abuse relatively quickly, emerge from their fear and anxiety, and get on with the rest of their lives.

The following case illustrates how going through the body can resolve the structural and emotional issues underlying anxiety.

Matthew: Freed from Fear and Anxiety

Matthew, 34, was plagued by fear, anxiety, and obsessive-compulsive tendencies. For most of his life, he had held the belief that he was going to die young and as a result was just waiting to die, although he wasn't conscious of living this way. Later he uncovered the fear that lay beneath this state, which was that he was convinced that there was something terribly wrong with him, that he had a terminal illness.

At the same time, he felt great anxiety over trying to make it in the world and worried about his survival. Fears about his survival filled his dreams as well. For as long as he could remember, he had had a recurrent nightmare of a plane crashing near him, with him having to run for his life and barely escaping the explosion from the crash. In waking life, he had the feeling of being trapped, unable to exert his will. An extreme fear arose, accompanied by nausea, when he was spinning or in an upside-down position. He also had deep anxiety and overwhelming feelings of inadequacy regarding sexual intercourse. This led to a constant fear of abandonment by his wife.

Matthew's obsessive-compulsiveness compelled him to complete tasks in a specified order, even when it was inefficient to do it that way. When he was prevented from observing this order, he felt "blocked in his head." He also reported feeling a cloudiness in his head at all times; this sensation had been with him for as long as he could remember.

His primary physical complaints were headaches, facial dermatitis, and digestive problems. He suffered from severe gas and had loose bowels 40 percent of the time. About twice a month, he would have an emergency-type bowel movement, where he had to run to make it to the toilet in time.

Two years before coming to Soma Therapy Centre, he had developed a tremor in his right arm and hand that made it difficult for him to write. His right arm also didn't swing when he walked. Matthew worked in a hospital and his father was a doctor, so he was medically knowledgeable. The tremor suggested to him early onset multiple sclerosis or Parkinson's disease, which only increased his anxiety. Fearing the worst, he did not consult a doctor, despite pressure from his family.

While Matthew had lived for decades with his anxiety and was able to keep it hidden, the physical symptom of the tremor was something he couldn't hide, and he had to do something about it. Deep down, he believed that the cause of the tremor was emotional, but seeking an explanation in the physical realm, he went to a chiropractor, who could find nothing organically wrong. He noted, however, that Matthew evidenced extreme anxiety during cervical (neck) and thoracic (upper back) adjustments. When six treatments produced no improvement in Matthew's symptoms, the chiropractor referred him to Soma Therapy Centre. He felt that there was an inner problem that needed to be addressed, which confirmed Matthew's unexpressed belief.

Soma therapy examination revealed that the components of the terrible triad were operative in Matthew. One factor was that the joint between his sphenoid, occipital, and temporal bones (this joint is known as the sphenobasilar symphysis) was compressed.

The sphenobasilar symphysis (SBS) is the cranial base, explains Steiner. "Unlike the top of the head, or vault, the base is not adaptive; it is structural. The ramifications of a compression of the SBS are that the rest of the cranium and the body have to adapt to it." In Matthew's case, not only did he have the back-to-front compression of the SBS, he also had the vertical misalignment of the occiput and sphenoid bones (the underlying vertical strain). The spinal cord enters the cranium in this area, as do major blood vessels, so the compressions and misalignments in Matthew's skull had further implications for his nervous and circulatory systems.

Matthew also evidenced misalignments in his upper neck vertebrae, which compromise the immune system and the limbic system (implicated in anxiety, as discussed in chapter 1) and affect chewing ability, among other consequences, states Steiner. The misalignment also produced restriction in his esophagus, which contributed to both his digestive problems and the sensations of anxiety.

Examination further revealed a brain spasm, which was likely the result of an impact injury, Steiner says. With a brain spasm, "there is a loss of fluid flow, as there is a hemorrhage that occurs in that area, and there is also often an emotional component related to the injury."

Finally, Matthew's examination showed that he had a loss of tissue vitality throughout his body from poor blood circulation and impaired nervous system function caused by the long-standing compression, explains Steiner. In Matthew's case, "the loss of the tissue vitality subtly and subliminally contributed to his sense of despair and doom, as he intrinsically felt and likely inherently perceived his body to be failing and shutting down."

Matthew's history revealed that he had indeed sustained impact injuries to his head. Two accidents he had when he was little were sufficient to explain all of his structural problems. One accident, which he knew about, happened when he was ten years old. He suffered a concussion after being pushed down at school in the wintertime and hitting his head hard on the ice. It took him five days to recover from the concussion. The other incident, the memory of which emerged during one of his sessions at Soma Therapy Centre, occurred when he was three months old. He was in a waiting room with his father and fell out of his infant chair, hitting his head.

"At three months, his cranial base would not have been really solid cartilage yet," notes Steiner. If Matthew had gotten a CranioSacral or cranial osteopathic adjustment after each of these falls, a good portion of his later problems could have been avoided. This is not to say that he wouldn't have developed an anxiety disorder, because there were strong emotional components in his case, but at least he wouldn't have had the exacerbation of structural issues as well. This serves as a good reminder to parents to seek this kind of treatment for their children if they suffer a blow to the head in a fall or other accident.

Without treatment, these two injuries led to severe compromise of the nervous system. For a long time, his body did a good job of compensating, "but eventually it became fatigued, began to lose ground, and finally could no longer compensate for the misalignment and compression," says Steiner. "When a nerve is stimulated, initially it is hyperexcitable [in an overexcited state] and then it goes into a state of hypoexcitability [reacting less than is normal]; it has been overstimulated to the point that it is no longer reactive." Matthew's right arm tremor was a manifestation of his failing nervous system.

In addition, Steiner says, "He was getting a message internally that he was shutting down. Whether or not he knew that consciously, the fact that he was not getting the same amount of neural stimulation and vascular flow [flow of blood through the blood vessels], on some level, is going to tell you that you're fragile. It's going to give you a sense of yourself that supports the growing anxiety." This likely related to Matthew's general state of anxiety and his fear that he was going to die.

Over the next 15 months, Matthew had 35 treatments (a combination of CranioSacral Therapy/SER, Visceral Manipulation, and Process Oriented Counseling) at Soma Therapy Centre. These treatments were initiated by Matthew. Clients are not automatically rescheduled for follow-up appointments at the Centre. "People know when they need to come back, based on their symptoms," explains Steiner. In this way, people take full responsibility for their own recovery. This is "healthy health care."

In Matthew's case, some of his appointment scheduling was anxiety based. "There were times when he booked in for a treatment because his wife felt that he should be moving through his process faster, and he was trying to comply." Matthew's commitment to his recovery, however, was strong on its own, apart from his wife. "When he became symptomatic, he understood that he needed to do another piece of work, and he would come in," says Steiner. "He started listening to his body."

Initially, Matthew's anxiety level during treatment was extreme. Lying on the treatment table, he would ask over and over, "Am I going to be able to move after this treatment? Am I going to be paralyzed? Am I going to die?" As he felt better after treatment, this in-session anxiety began to subside.

Emotional content emerged during many of his treatments, and memories that helped explain his fear and anxiety surfaced in Matthew. During one treatment, which was focusing on his head and neck, he relived his birth, including hearing his mother talk with the doctor. It was clear by the conversation that she suffered from fears and anxiety (hypochondria) similar to his own.

In other sessions, memories surfaced from his early childhood of being sexually abused by a friend of his father's and, later, by his father. Feelings of terror, being trapped, and fear that he was dying flooded him as these emotions were released from his body tissue. During this time, Matthew and his wife went into couple's counseling. Later, he joined a support group for male survivors of sexual abuse and then started individual counseling.

Matthew reported that his fears and anxieties decreased dramatically after the first memories of abuse. This raises an important point regarding the work done at Soma Therapy Centre. Some people express scepticism that anyone can remember what happened during their birth or when they were two years old or when they were in the womb. But the fact that a person's symptoms improve dramatically or disappear after release of traumatic events confirms that the trauma happened and that it contributed to the person's condition.

In Matthew's case, the reduction in his lifetime anxiety came only after release of the abuse memories. "The improvements are what told him that the abuse was true," recalls Steiner. "It becomes relatively undeniable. If having that recollection releases you from the grip of fear, then how can you deny it? That's the nature of this work. People go back and get memories of conception or three months old or whatever, and all of that is just as deniable as the memory of sexual abuse, but how can you deny it when the effect on your physical being and your emotional being as an adult is so profound?"

The results also support the concept of cellular memory, the body as a repository of memories of which the person may not be consciously aware. It is clear from the soma therapy process and the outcome that something is released from the body, whether the process sparks specific recollection of past trauma or not.

Matthew's anxiety over his sexual performance decreased after he realized that it was connected to the abuse. He recognized that the anxiety was not about what was happening in the present moment, but was a reenactment of the abuse. His fear of abandonment had similar roots. Seeing this, he was less controlled by that fear. When he discovered that it wasn't possible for him to heal from the abuse in the context of his marriage, he was able to let go. He and his wife ended their marriage, but remained good friends.

Matthew's obsessive-compulsive disorder (OCD) began to disappear after a treatment session in which he recognized that doing things one at a time in a rigid order was connected to the brain injury he had sustained at three months old. The OCD behaviors were a neurological compensation for the damage to his system. After that recognition (treatment had also corrected the structural misalignments and compressions), he reported that he was able to multi-task, something that had been almost impossible for him before.

Treatment at Soma Therapy Centre resulted in a resolution of his digestive problems, headaches, and brain fog as well. Matthew reports that his dermatitis still comes and goes. He has made the link that outbreaks are "totally related" to feelings he is not expressing. As soon as he gets in touch with these feelings, the dermatitis clears up.

As for the tremor in his arm and hand, he still has it, but it is much better and he has regained much of his dexterity. Previously, his palm was often clammy; this disappeared in the course of treatment.

As the tremor was not entirely gone, Matthew finally went to see a neurologist. The result had an ironic twist. Medical examination revealed no organic source for the tremor, and the neurologist concurred that emotional trauma was the cause.

While Matthew's intuition that he needed to look to the emotions in order to resolve the tremor was correct, there was also neurological recovery that had to happen because of his untreated injuries and the effect they had on the nervous system. With the structural problems from those injuries corrected, Matthew could focus on the final pieces of his emotional recovery. "I know now," he says, "that I am afraid to be fully in my body. I need to regain equilibrium within my survival responses. My body is stuck in surrender." He continues to work on his emotional healing but does not feel that he has to wait until he is fully healed before he gets on with his life. "My life can move forward, with the last of the residual trauma coming into awareness and getting handled when it does."

Matthew has learned how to access his memories himself, how to work with them, and how not to be afraid of what comes up. Now, when he has the occasional disturbing dream or waking memory, it no longer sends him into a panic.

8 Energy, Trauma, and Spirit: Thought Field Therapy and Seemorg Matrix Work

When it comes to anxiety, "talk" therapy is a primary treatment (along with antianxiety medications) conventionally associated with the condition. While we have seen in this book that many factors that cause anxiety are not addressed by such therapy, we have also seen that psychospiritual issues frequently play a role and may need to be attended to for long-lasting resolution of the condition. This chapter explores two psychotherapeutic techniques: Thought Field Therapy (TFT) and Seemorg Matrix Work.

Rather than focusing on verbal processing of psychospiritual issues, these methods are energy-based psychotherapies. Their operating premise is that disturbances in an individual's energy field underlie anxiety, panic attacks, phobia, addiction, depression, and other symptoms and conditions. Such disturbances can be caused by "energy toxins" or psychospiritual trauma. By clearing the energy field, resolution of the condition can be achieved. These methods are much faster than standard psychotherapy, and they address the underlying energy problems, which standard forms do not.

Tony Roffers, Ph.D., of Oakland, California, has been a psychotherapist for more than 30 years and has expertise in a range of psychotherapeutic modalities. In recent years, he began using

Thought Field Therapy and Seemorg Matrix Work and was so impressed by the results that they are now the centerpieces of his practice. In the case of Seemorg Matrix Work, Dr. Roffers works closely with the founder of the method and is the most versed practitioner, aside from her, worldwide. Hundreds of therapists have been trained in both of these techniques as word of their effectiveness has spread. The particular specialty of Thought Field Therapy is in treating anxiety disorders.

More about Thought Field Therapy

As discussed in chapter 3, Thought Field Therapy (TFT) works in the body's Thought Field (the Mental Body in Dr. Klinghardt's model). Blocked or disturbed energy flow in this field is corrected through tapping on certain acupuncture points on the body while the client thinks of the situations, events, or objects that trigger the distress. TFT is well known for its ability to relieve anxiety, phobias, and panic attacks and to do so quickly and often permanently. Sometimes, all it takes is a five-minute treatment, which clients (including children) can learn to do themselves in the event of a return of symptoms.

Dr. Roffers has found TFT to be most effective for phobias, quick reduction of anxiety, relieving the symptoms of posttraumatic stress disorder (PTSD), and some forms of depression. He uses TFT in crisis situations, instances in which you need "quick results."

The operating principle of TFT is that anxiety and other disorders are manifestations of an energy perturbation in the acupuncture meridian system (see chapters 3 and 4). In other words, some disturbance has thrown your energy system out of whack. Clinical psychologist Roger J. Callahan, Ph.D., the founder of TFT, was a pioneer in cognitive therapy, a form of "talk" therapy that focuses on retraining the mind out of old patterns in order to produce emotional and behavioral changes. His research and clinical experience led him to rethink his approach, however, and the result was TFT.

"Many experts in the mental health field today believe that chemistry or cognitions are the fundamental cause of disturbed emotions," states Dr. Callahan. "The basic premise of Thought Field Therapy, however, is that the perturbation(s) in the thought field precedes and generates these chemical and cognitive facts."[175] The response of patients to TFT supports the energy model. Dr. Callahan claims a 75 to 80 percent success rate, meaning that "75 to 80 percent of people can expect to have their negative emotions completely resolved."[176]

In one independent study of people with posttraumatic stress disorder, symptoms in the 34 subjects decreased by nearly 40 percent after one treatment, and 18 of the 34 improved to the point that they no longer met PTSD diagnostic criteria.[177]

According to the TFT model, the perturbations, or disturbances, in the energy field often result from energy toxins, or allergies, sensitivities, or intolerances, as they are variously termed. The phrase "energy toxin" reflects how the offending substance can throw the energy system out of balance. Heavy metal toxicities fall into the category of energy toxins as well.

Both the TFT and Matrix Work models recognize that psychological trauma can also create energy perturbations. "Traumatic experiences in childhood, in the womb, even in past lives or in your heritage, can be the source of aberrations in your energy field," explains Dr. Roffers.

Both the TFT and Matrix Work models recognize that psychological trauma can also create energy perturbations. "Traumatic experiences in childhood, in the womb, even in past lives or in your heritage, can be the source of aberrations in your energy field," explains Dr. Roffers.

In TFT, it is not necessary to determine the cause of the energy aberration or gain insight into your anxiety, as is the traditional approach in psychotherapy. "The only insight you need is that there was something messed up in your meridians that has now been fixed, and you now know how to fix it on your own if you need to."

In Their Own Words

"I'm 36 years old and I'm afraid to cross streets by myself. . . .I had a really important appointment. . . . I got out of the taxi not worrying about a thing until I saw that I was on the wrong side of Sixth Avenue. There was no way I could cross that street."[178]

—a man who suffered from a phobia of crossing streets

In many cases, a quick TFT treatment is all it takes to correct the energy problem and eliminate the anxiety. If TFT doesn't work, it is typically because something you are eating, breathing, or being exposed to reinstates the energy perturbation, or an early trauma that has not been uncovered or treated is keeping the energy problem in place, explains Dr. Roffers. In these cases, allergy identification and elimination techniques such as NAET (see chapters 2 and 3) and psychotherapeutic methods such as Seemorg Matrix Work (see below) may be necessary to resolve the disturbance.

A classic example of the kind of case for which TFT is "incredibly effective," says Dr. Roffers, is the roofer who suddenly has a panic attack while working on a roof because he suddenly finds himself afraid of heights. If he used his cell phone to call a TFT practitioner, that person could instruct him on the points to tap, and "in three to nine minutes he could be back to working on the roof—literally." The roofer does not know why he had the attack, but it is gone. "Many people really are not interested and don't care where those awful feelings came from," he notes. They just want to get rid of them.

This runs counter to the approach of the majority of traditional psychotherapists, Dr. Roffers observes, which is why many regard TFT as not a true therapy because it doesn't lead to understanding or insight that could have application to other aspects of the client's life. "The notion that insight is a necessary prerequisite for behavioral change is a very strong notion in Western psychology," he states. "I personally have gone through quite a transformation about that, in the sense that I think insight is often an important prerequisite and does aid in the generalization of therapeutic work to other arenas of the client's life, but I no longer see it as a necessary prerequisite.

"Insight assumes that the mind, one's awareness, can really influence one's behavior and can lead you to the heart of the matter," Dr. Roffers says, but according to Thought Field Therapy, "it's really a perturbation in the thought field that's at the heart of the matter. This perturbation serves as a trigger for all kinds of aberrations that are on neurological, hormonal, chemical, and cognitive levels." In other words, an energy disturbance can produce all kinds of physical and mental symptoms, and if you resolve the issue in the energy field, the symptoms go away.

This raises the question: if your anxiety can be resolved in five minutes, why would you bother with a psychotherapeutic method that takes longer?

To return to the example of the roofer, the Matrix Work model holds that "if you just treated his fear of heights on that roof, it would more than likely come up in other areas and in other ways, and we need to find whatever the originating traumas were that caused that panic attack on the roof," explains Dr. Roffers. On the other hand, the TFT model holds that this may or may not be true; in many cases, clearing the energy perturbation is all it takes.

Dr. Roffers has found that the more traumas you have, the more you have to use TFT around the different aspects of the trauma. "If in fact the roofer had a number of different traumatic experiences, either on his job as a roofer or when he was a child, it is likely he would need a lot of different treatments for different aspects or types of traumatic experiences," he explains.

Among his clients, Dr. Roffers has encountered both situations—those whose anxiety is resolved quickly and does not return and those who need deeper exploration. As an example of the latter, he cites the case of an attorney who developed a phobia of going into the courtroom after he failed in his representation of two jury cases. He came to Dr. Roffers because he was unable to face going back into the courtroom. The TFT treatment for anxiety around the jury experiences and his unwillingness to enter into another jury trial didn't work. After trying many different tapping combinations or formulas (called algorithms) to alleviate the anxiety, Dr. Roffers discovered that underlying the anxiety was depression, which cleared very quickly with TFT treatment.

The anxiety still did not resolve, however, and Dr. Roffers and the client are now doing Matrix Work, uncovering early trauma that relates to the issue of failure, which created the energy blockage. "He's still not back in the courtroom, but we've gotten further using the Matrix Work methods. In other words, in my experience, TFT has not been a panacea for all things." For deeper insight and clearing of the issues underlying anxiety or other disorders, Dr. Roffers relies on Matrix Work.

For help locating a TFT practitioner, contact the Callahan Techniques office, 78-816 Via Carmel, La Quinta, CA 92253; tel: 760-564-1008; website: www.tftrx.com (professional site), www.self helpuniv.com (self-help site). For information about Seemorg Matrix Work, contact Asha Nahoma Clinton, Ph.D., Energy Revolution, Inc., 885 East Rd., Richmond, MA 01254; tel: 413-698-2744; e-mail: energyrev@seemorgmatrix.org; website: www.seemorgmatrix.org. The website has a directory of practitioners.

What Is *Seemorg Matrix Work*?

Psychotherapist Asha Nahoma Clinton, L.C.S.W., Ph.D., developed Seemorg Matrix Work in the mid-1990s as a result of her dissatisfaction with the results produced by psychodynamic psychotherapy, which she had been practicing for 20 years. Matrix Work is "the first transpersonal, body-centered energy psychotherapy," states Dr. Clinton. "It treats trauma and its many psychological, physical, intellectual, and spiritual aftereffects with the movement of energy through the major energy centers."[179]

The transpersonal psychotherapy aspect of Seemorg Matrix Work is found in its focus on "removing the blocks that impede spiritual development" and "a spiritual technology to nurture and enhance that development."[180]

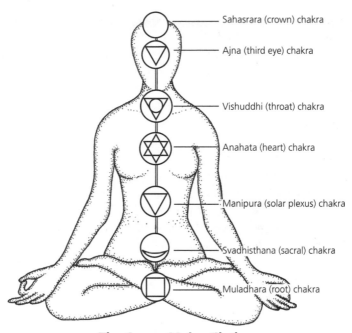

Sahasrara (crown) chakra

Ajna (third eye) chakra

Vishuddhi (throat) chakra

Anahata (heart) chakra

Manipura (solar plexus) chakra

Svadhisthana (sacral) chakra

Muladhara (root) chakra

The Seven Major Chakras

Its name reflects this orientation; Seemorg (a variation on Simorgh), a fabulous bird featured in Persian and Indian tales, is a symbol of the Divine.[181]

The major energy centers to which Dr. Clinton refers are the chakras, the series of seven energy vortexes positioned along the midline of the body from the base of the spine to the crown of the head. As discussed in chapter 3, when chakras are blocked, the free flow of energy in the body's field is impeded. Matrix Work uses the chakra system, progressing from top to bottom, to move negative energy out of the body. It then proceeds through the chakras from bottom to top, bringing positive energy into the body. This is the body-centered energy aspect of the therapy.

Dr. Roffers, who, as noted previously, works closely with Dr. Clinton, explains the relevance of the chakras to psychotherapy: "The chakras are like switchboards for the meridian system, central energy centers for this electromagnetic circulatory system in the body.

Seemorg Matrix Work is a way of working with your energy system that can put it back into alignment." According to Dr. Clinton's model, trauma is the source of aberrations in a person's energy field, and those aberrations produce mind and body disorders.

There are essentially two kinds of traumas, says Dr. Roffers. One is the crisis type of trauma, as in your father beat you or you fell off the garage roof. The other is developmental trauma, which is more subtle and occurs over a period of time. The experience of having a distant father or a critical mother is an example of developmental trauma. Dr. Clinton's therapy works with the energy system to clear those traumas in your body on an energetic level. With the traumas cleared and the energy balance restored, the disorders that stemmed from the energy aberration can self-correct.

The Matrix approach works in "a much more holistic, integrated way than the traditional talking therapy," states Dr. Roffers. It also significantly reduces the healing time, although it is still not a quick fix. "The metaphor I use is if you're going to remodel your kitchen and someone starts going into the walls and finds out where a leak is, pretty soon the whole kitchen may be torn apart."

Matrix Work can be effective in the traditionally difficult areas of multiple diagnosis, dissociation, and personality disorder, as well as with issues that are less complex, according to Dr. Clinton. The therapy can also be used to clear energy toxins (allergies). As discussed in chapter 2, allergies can be an underlying factor in anxiety.

According to the Seemorg Matrix model, trauma is at the root of many allergies; the hypothesis is that the substance was in the person's energy field when the trauma occurred, and so the person developed "disharmony" with that substance. The disharmony can be reversed by reintroducing the substance into the person's field and using Matrix Work to move through all the chakras, removing the aftereffects of trauma and realigning the energy.

Dr. Roffers notes that regardless of how the allergy began, whether the hypothesis holds true or not, "aligning the meridians and the chakras in this way strengthens the person's system, aligns them, or puts them more in harmony with whatever the substance is." He adds, "I'm getting better results clearing energy toxins using Matrix Work, and specifically the clearing of traumas, than with any of the other methods I've used." Dr. Roffers is trained in several other energy-based allergy elimination techniques.

"Modern-Day Exorcism"

Dr. Roffers calls Matrix Work "modern-day exorcism." This is a reference to the legitimate and effective energy work that exorcism, as performed by skilled shamans of old, entailed (and still entails; see chapter 9). Matrix Work removes the energy influences to which we are subject today.

The work begins with the practitioner taking a thorough history, including what is known as a "trauma history." For the latter, clients list whatever traumas, of both the crisis and developmental types, they can remember.

To monitor the status of energy in the body throughout the work that follows, the therapist uses kinesiological muscle testing. For this, you hold one arm straight out in front of you and attempt to keep it there while the practitioner pushes down slightly on your arm. Normally, you can easily hold your arm in place, but when there is an energy disturbance in your meridian system, the muscle response is weakened. While you are being tested, the practitioner has you think of the trauma or asks you to make specific statements.

First, however, the practitioner tests you to make sure that you are not "neurologically disorganized." Other terms or phrases for this condition are "switched," being in "massive reversal," or having your polarization off, states Dr. Roffers. Regardless of the term, the upshot is that if you are in this state, muscle testing will not be reliable.

To check for neurological disorganization, you place either hand on top of your head with the palm down, then extend your other arm out in front of you for the practitioner to test as in the standard muscle testing, Dr. Roffers explains. If the arm tests strong, the body is in alignment. When you turn the palm of the hand on your head up instead of down, the extended arm should test weak, because that position takes the body out of alignment. Any other combination (such as when the palm is down, the arm is weak; or when the palm is up, the arm is strong) is a reversal, a sign of neurological disorganization. The practitioner must then use a technique to realign the person so muscle testing will be accurate.

The next step in the Matrix process is the Covenant. The therapist starts by asking the client to say, "I give permission for my being to be healed." If the arm response on that is weak, it means the person is not giving permission. "You have to clear that or they're not ready to be treated," Dr. Roffers states. "By clearing any negative beliefs that get in the way of treating traumas, the Covenant is a way of assuring that the person is going to be open to the treatment and, once you treat traumas, that those treatments will hold."

To clear the negative belief, you hold a hand over each chakra in turn, going from top to bottom, repeating the belief at each chakra. The therapist then conducts the muscle testing again to make sure that the negative statement has cleared from the body. A positive belief about the treatment (for example, "I can be healed") is then instilled in the same way, but by going up the chakras, from bottom to top.

While one hand moves from chakra to chakra, the other maintains a position over the primary chakra for that particular person. "The primary chakra is the energy center that has been most adversely affected by the trauma the client needs to clear," Dr. Roffers explains. In his experience, for traumas, many people need to hold the heart chakra, but it can be the solar plexus or another chakra. For negative beliefs, the primary chakra is usually the third-eye point (sixth chakra) on the forehead.

To determine an individual's primary chakra, Dr. Roffers has the person hold one hand over a chakra while he does muscle testing on the person's other arm. A strong response indicates that it is the primary chakra. A weak response indicates the need to test the next chakra and continue until the primary chakra is identified.

The primary chakra is called the stationary point. The client keeps one hand on the primary chakra throughout the process. "The two hands create an electromagnetic loop," he explains. "My hypothesis is that by closing that electromagnetic loop, you're realigning something in the body that's been misaligned and, as you clear that loop, something shifts. Then when you go to the next level, something else shifts." You will find that some chakras don't have any misalignment in them, he adds.

After the Covenant is completed, the therapist moves to

clearing traumas, first identifying the primary chakra (stationary point) and a phrase that describes the trauma (for example, "My father abandoned me"). The client then moves down through the chakras, repeating the phrase at each.

There is no rigid order in proceeding with Seemorg Matrix Work because it is tailored to the client, notes Dr. Roffers, but generally the focus at this point turns to the originating traumas. These are the traumas that occurred very early in life. To clarify the nature of trauma, Dr. Clinton offers the following definition:

"A trauma is any occurrence which, when we think of it or it is triggered by some present event, evokes difficult emotions and/or physical symptoms; gives rise to negative beliefs, desire, fantasies, compulsions, obsessions, addictions or dissociation; blocks the development of positive qualities and spiritual connection; and fractures human wholeness."[182]

After working with the originating traumas, the focus shifts to the initiatory traumas, usually the events that brought the person into therapy. "These are the much more recent traumas," explains Dr. Roffers, "which are a retraumatization of the originating traumas."

The next step is to clear traumatic patterns. These are like a web of traumas that gets woven around an originating trauma; you could also call this web a syndrome of traumas. For example, "if you had a very cold and distant father, you selectively attend to men who are that way, and you begin to attract men who are cold and distant, as a misguided attempt to heal," says Dr. Roffers. The belief, "All men are cold and distant," is formed secondarily as a result of the originating and subsequent traumas.

The next step is to clear the negative or dysfunctional beliefs that have accrued as a result of traumas and instill the more positive or functional beliefs using the Core Belief Matrix. "A matrix is a cluster of interrelated core beliefs around a certain trauma," explains Dr. Roffers. A Core Belief Matrix is a series of statements, stated first in the negative and then in the positive, that reflect core beliefs. An example of a negative statement in a Matrix is "I can be used," while the corresponding positive statement is "I will no longer permit being used."

The client says each negative statement in turn, with the

therapist conducting muscle testing. When a person says "I can be used" and the arm response is strong, it means the person believes that statement. Before proceeding to the next statement, "you have to take that dysfunctional belief out," says Dr. Roffers. The client goes down the chakras, saying the negative core belief. Then the corresponding positive core belief—"I will no longer permit being used"—is instilled by going up the chakras, repeating the positive statement at each chakra with one hand placed on the third-eye chakra (between the eyes) as the stationary point.

By clearing the traumas, traumatic patterns, and negative core beliefs and realigning the attendant energy imbalance, a condition such as anxiety can be resolved. As with other energy-based modalities, correcting the energy flow often results in self-correction of factors that present in anxiety and may seem to be the cause, such as hormonal or neurotransmitter imbalances.

As stated previously, another corollary of Seemorg Matrix Work is that it tends to open people up to spiritual possibilities. "To me, it's a major answer to how psychological work integrates with spiritual development," says Dr. Roffers. "If you have trauma, it separates you from God. It separates you from yourself. It separates you from others. It separates you from the Earth, the universe."

Clearing traumas and the self-sabotaging negative beliefs that cluster around them enables you "to become more whole within yourself, and you're much more open and permeable and interested in working on that spiritual level." Having worked extensively with the Matrix method, Dr. Roffers now believes that this clearing can be done for most people and for most types of trauma.

The following case history from Dr. Roffers' files demonstrates how Thought Field Therapy and Matrix Work can be used in combination to resolve anxiety.

Melissa: Anxiety and Relationships

Melissa came to Dr. Roffers when she was in her mid-twenties because of the severe anxiety she experienced whenever she was in a relationship. Each time she got involved with a man, she became emotionally dependent on him. When he chose to do something without her, she "freaked out." Naturally, this put great stress on her relationships. When her partner talked about breaking up, as he inevitably did, she became "incredibly anxious," to the point of panic. This had been her pattern since she had begun having boyfriends.

When Dr. Roffers first started working with Melissa, it was before he had discovered TFT and Matrix Work. His psychotherapeutic approach was more traditional and emphasized cognitive-behavioral therapy (CBT). In the course of their sessions, Melissa made important connections between her pattern with men and the fact that her father had left her mother and the family two or three times during her childhood. He would leave in the middle of the night without her knowing it, and she would only find out the next morning after he was gone. The period before he left would be characterized by intense battles between her parents.

It was clear that there was much in her history to account for her current difficulties, states Dr. Roffers. In their sessions, they did "a lot of relationship therapy and cognitive work around her dysfunctional belief that every man would do what her father did."

As a result of this work, which occurred over a period of several years, Melissa was able to function better in her intimate relationships. While she no longer "freaked out" when the man did something independently or got overinvolved in his work, she had a tendency to become demanding or clingy at these times, and her relationships still didn't last long. Whenever she faced a breakup, the level of anxiety she felt was still high, although it had decreased some.

Where formerly it was at nine on a scale of ten, with ten being extreme panic attacks, it was now at six or seven, notes Dr. Roffers. Melissa, who no longer felt she needed ongoing therapy, would come back for help in getting through the breakup. Despite all her insights, her anxiety level at these times wasn't down to a manageable level.

Meanwhile, Dr. Roffers had begun using TFT, so when Melissa faced yet another breakup, he was able to use this technique with her. During the tapping, he had her focus on her current anxiety and in another sequence, on her father leaving. "We were able to deal with her anxiety around the breakup easier, faster, and better with the TFT."

At the same time as he initiated the TFT, Dr. Roffers had Melissa reduce her sugar and alcohol intake. He has found that these high-glycemic carbohydrates tend to disrupt treatment and are often implicated as energy toxins in cases of anxiety. Such clients are often hypersensitive to these substances. They suffer from hypoglycemia (low blood sugar), which means that these substances send them on a roller coaster of rapidly rising then plummeting glucose (blood sugar) levels. "This seems to be very highly correlated with anxiety," he notes.

Melissa reduced her intake significantly but was able to have sugar or alcohol occasionally without detrimental effects. In her case, these things exacerbated her anxiety but were not the originating cause.

She had five or six TFT sessions over two months to clear the many traumas related to her father leaving the family unannounced and the later retraumatization from being left by numerous boyfriends. Her anxiety decreased, although it was not entirely resolved. She made more progress in those two months of TFT, however, than she had in the years of traditional psychotherapy, observes Dr. Roffers. It is important to note though that the degree to which that earlier work helped to make TFT treatment simpler is unknown. So Melissa could alleviate her anxiety if it returned, Dr. Roffers taught her how to do the tapping.

Melissa was entering a new relationship at the time of her last breakup. After the TFT work, she found that she had more control over her anxiety at occurrences that would have triggered panic before, such as when her partner had to travel for business, and she was able to manage day-to-day life with him much better too. In fact, the relationship went so well that they got engaged.

It was not relationship trouble that brought Melissa back to Dr. Roffers, but two car accidents that retriggered the trauma of an earlier event. During the earlier period of her more traditional psychotherapy, a highly upsetting incident had occurred. In her car one night, she was at a stop sign when someone suddenly smashed the car window with a brick and stole her purse before she even realized what was going on. A lot of glass rained in upon her, and she felt the incident as a traumatic invasion. It was hard for her to drive after that, especially at night, but through therapy and later TFT, she released most of the anxiety and was able to drive again.

Now, some years later, Melissa had gotten into two automobile accidents within a short time and was having trouble driving again. This time, Dr. Roffers suggested Seemorg Matrix Work, which he had begun using in his practice since her last visit, and Melissa readily agreed.

She rated her anxiety level while driving at seven or eight on the scale of ten. When Dr. Roffers did muscle testing to check the old traumatic incident of having her car window smashed and her purse stolen, the anxiety had gone up somewhat from the last time they had dealt with it. Melissa gave her anxiety a subjective rating of three or four, and Dr. Roffers corroborated this with the muscle testing. The first of her two recent accidents tested at eight and the second at ten.

Dr. Roffers then used Matrix Work to clear the energy blockages in her body, and thus her anxiety. He instructed her to think about the original robbery incident, while holding her stationary hand on the heart chakra and using her other hand to go down through the chakras. That procedure brought her anxiety down to a zero within two to three minutes, and Melissa reported that the anxiety over the incident felt distant. "She certainly had the memory of the event, but she didn't have the emotional charge around it. The anxiety, in essence, was gone."

They then turned to the first of the two recent accidents, which was more like an initiatory trauma, notes Dr. Roffers. "We had to go through three traumatic aspects of that one." The first was when, out of the corner of her eye, she saw the car that hit her coming at her; the second was when the car hit her; and a third came when she was standing on the traffic island in the rain, looking at her car and the traffic going around it. "Each of these we matrixed; we went down the chakras for each aspect of the trauma, with her thinking of each. In about 20 minutes, she was no longer feeling any anxiety. It was a zero."

The second accident was similar, though she had been with her fiancé that time and it had been a more intense trauma. Again, there were two or three different components or aspects to clear. One of them was that the car hit on her fiancé's side and raised the fear that she would lose him. Dr. Roffers tested to see if there was a connection between that and her father and there was. So after getting the anxiety about the other aspects of the accident down to zero, they turned to doing Matrix Work around her issues with her father.

Matrix Work unpeeled the final layer of Melissa's anxiety, cleared the related negative core beliefs and installed positive core beliefs to support her well-being in a relationship, and released her from the energy disturbances and early traumas that had been dictating her emotions and behavior.

All of this was accomplished in one session. In a second session, scheduled for follow-up, Melissa reported that she was feeling fine and had been able to drive without a recurrence of her anxiety. "She said she had the memory of feeling anxious and was worried about getting anxious, but it wasn't there, which is often the case," Dr. Roffers notes.

They spent the session matrixing her father issues. Melissa wanted to work on that because she wished to get married and was concerned about her issues interfering with her relationship again. It was clear that the intense anxiety that arose in her during a breakup had its roots in her father leaving without telling her. In Matrix Work, they uncovered a primary core belief connected to that, which was: "If I have a man in my life, he of necessity will leave or die." Another core belief, which was operational in the car accident with her fiancé, was: "When things are going good, something bad's going to happen."

"Those beliefs are the way we perpetuate our traumas in our

current life," says Dr. Roffers. "Even when the trauma is clear, if we still have that belief, we keep the trauma alive. And it can create a self-fulfilling prophecy." To truly clear the trauma, it is necessary to clear the core belief as well. In Melissa's case, if Matrix Work hadn't cleared the belief regarding the inevitability of something bad happening, "she might have continued her life thinking that the better the marriage got, the more sure it was that she was going to lose him prematurely."

As it was, Matrix Work unpeeled the final layer of Melissa's anxiety, cleared the related negative core beliefs and installed positive core beliefs to support her well-being in a relationship, and released her from the energy disturbances and early traumas that had been dictating her emotions and behavior. At a two-years follow-up, Melissa reported that she is happily married and able to function normally when her husand leaves on business or personal trips. She also no longer has that feeling of impending doom when things are going well.

9 Psychic and Shamanic Healing

While psychic healing and shamanic healing may seem to be in an entirely different category from the other therapies covered in this book, they are actually other forms of holistic medicine. Like homeopathy, they address disturbances in an individual's electromagnetic or energy field and, in so doing, bring body, mind, and spirit back into alignment. While each energy-based therapy has its own method for dealing with energy disturbances, the goal is the same: the clearing of negative influences and blockages, and the restoration of balance, wholeness, and connectedness.

The negative influences and blockages addressed by psychic and shamanic healing are found in the energy field that surrounds the body, which is also called the aura. While, unlike psychics and shamans, laypeople cannot typically see their aura, they receive evidence of its existence all the time. Have you ever "felt your skin crawl" when you met someone new? Have you ever suddenly and for no apparent reason felt drained or depressed when you walked into a room of people? These reactions are the result of discordant foreign energies entering your energy field, or aura, where they are not a good match with your energy and consequently produce a sense of unease or discomfort.

Unfortunately, energy influences are not just transitory. The energy field around your body is subtle and fragile and can be damaged, which renders it more permeable to foreign energies and more likely that they will remain. Among the events or practices that can damage or pollute the aura are emotional or physical trauma, psychic or verbal abuse, other people's negative or bad thoughts about you, and substance abuse. Physicians and psychics alike have noted that the energy field can be poisoned or polluted by harmful energies that produce mental, emotional, and physical symptoms and, if allowed to remain, can lead to disease.[183]

Psychiatrist Shakuntala Modi, M.D., of Wheeling, West Virginia, has been researching energy field disturbances for more than 15 years. She has identified a range of physical and psychological symptoms and conditions that result from such disturbances, including panic disorders, depression, headaches, allergies, uterine disorders, weight gain, stammering, and schizophrenia. Further, under clinical hypnotherapy (a form of therapy that involves inducing a hypnotic, or trancelike, state in the patient in order to access the unconscious mind), 77 out of 100 patients cited foreign "beings" in their aura as responsible for the symptoms or condition for which they were pursuing treatment. Dr. Modi's research revealed that these beings (foreign energies) are "the single leading cause of psychiatric problems."[184] Dr. Modi also found that after removing the foreign energies from the patient's energy field using hypnotherapy, the patient's symptoms "often cleared up immediately."[185]

The concept of energy disturbances in a person's energy field causing a variety of physical and psychological problems is gaining greater recognition and acceptance in the healing professions and among the public at large. A simple way to look at the issue of "energy pollution" is that, like the environment and your body, your energy field is subject to toxic buildup and requires cleansing to restore it to health. Just as we take measures to clean up our planet and engage in various body detoxification methods such as fasts or colonics, we need to take steps to clear the toxins from our auras. Psychic and shamanic healing are methods for cleansing your energy field of the toxins that are interfering with your physical, emotional, and spiritual health.

Psychic Healing

Psychic healing involves the removal of foreign energy from your energy field, says Reverend Leon S. LeGant, of San Rafael,

California. He has been a clairvoyant all his life and has worked as a psychic healer for the past eight years, clearing hundreds of people of the disruptive influences in their energy fields. Now, as executive director of the Psychic School, a nonprofit organization dedicated to the development of psychic abilities, he is devoting much of his time to training others in this type of healing.

Simply put, a psychic is someone who is sensitive to non-physical forces. LeGant believes that everyone is psychic to some degree. Their abilities vary depending on when they shut themselves down, which most people do between the ages of three and five in response to parental and societal invalidation of the spirit realm, he says.

LeGant defines clairvoyance as "the ability to see energy in the form of mental image pictures. Since everything in the universe is made of energy, you can see it clairvoyantly in the form of a symbol or image or a picture that would make sense to the person seeing the information or the image." He notes that, without the proper context for the visions, clairvoyance is easily labeled hallucination.

Childhood fears of the dark, of monsters in the closet, of things under the bed actually have foundation in reality, arising as they do from children's "clairvoyance sensing an energy in the room with them." Since it is frightening, they begin to turn off their clairvoyance, explains LeGant. The programming of the educational system and usually their parents as well supports this suppression. "There's no validation for clairvoyance or being sensitive," he notes.

The imaginary friends of childhood also indicate children's connection to the spirit realm. These friends are their spirit guides. Again, messages from outside invalidate what children know to be true and teach them that "what they're sensing and seeing is not real, it's just an illusion or something they're making up." In most families, growing up requires that you stop having tea with your imaginary friends.

For some people, suppressing contact with the spirit realm is more difficult than for others. Psychics actually have "slightly different neurochemistry," LeGant explains. "Their pineal gland is usually a little larger, and there may be a genetic component to it that affect their brain chemistry and allows them to process energy in the form of images and thoughts in their mind." In adolescence, the brain chemistry shifts, and the clairvoyance becomes highly active again. It takes that amount of time for the body to develop and be able to receive the information. Around the time that the neurochemistry changes is when psychics become hypersensitive. They can easily be overwhelmed by everything they are taking in and all that they are feeling as a result. "It's a lot to process," says LeGant.

A "grounded psychic" can balance between the physical and spiritual worlds and distinguish them from each other, but few psychics are assisted in accomplishing this until they are adults and are fortunate enough to find the help they need in handling their abilities. This has implications for "mental" illness. While you as a person with an anxiety disorder may not identify as a psychic, at the very least you share with psychics the characteristic of hypersensitivity.

Anxiety and Foreign Energies

Anyone with a mental illness is being influenced on some level through their spiritual sensitivity, says LeGant. In the case of anxiety and depression, most who suffer from it are highly sensitive people. "They get overwhelmed with other people's emotions, other people's problems, other people's pain. They often get cut off from their own emotions because they're flooded with everyone else's. All this foreign energy gets absorbed into their body, into their aura, into their chakra system, and becomes a very heavy, weighted energy." Being overwhelmed in this way can lead to both anxiety and depression.

Becoming overwhelmed by foreign energy is especially likely to happen to healers. Psychotherapists, doctors, spiritual healers, and others in the healing profession "may not know how to handle another person's energy, so they end up absorbing their pain and their problems [i.e., foreign energy]. If they're absorbing someone else's problem into their space, that problem will start to attract matching problems to them in their own life. Then they're trying to solve that problem, but it was never *their* problem in the first place."

Pain is "stuck energy," and when you absorb it, it weighs you down. "Someone who gets that overwhelmed and flooded with foreign energy leaves their body," says LeGant. Regardless of the fact that the mind has checked out and is no longer aware of the foreign energy, the body continues to absorb others' pain (stuck energy), and its own energy flow becomes blocked. "An antianxiety drug or antidepressant helps in the sense that it shuts down the person's clairvoyance and sensitivity and they feel less overwhelmed, but the pain is still in their body." This is why after many people go off their medications and the chemical leaves their system, they become overwhelmed again. "It's because the pain's still there," states LeGant.

The Beings in Your Energy Field

Another component of anxiety in the psychic model is spirit attachment. To understand how this works, it is necessary to consider life forms in the dimensions beyond the third dimension in which we live.

"Fifth dimensional life forms are angels and the various beings of the angelic hierarchy. The fifth dimension is what most religions and forms of spirituality would consider heaven," explains LeGant. "The fourth dimension is the in-between world where lost souls go if they are disconnected from the Supreme Being or confused. For example, someone who has died and is in resistance toward leaving their family and moving on will be in this dimension."

The fourth dimension, which intersects our world, is home to a lot of "beings," which are energy life forms that could also be called spirits. There's a wide spectrum of beings, whose nature depends upon their evolution, LeGant says. "Some are just observers, just watching and not interfering; some are very nice, helpful healers; and some are very destructive, harmful, negative beings that will lead people into mental illness, from anxiety to depression to suicide to schizophrenia." They lead people into many other places as well. There's a being for almost everything, and the influence of their "dark energy" is responsible for the negative state of the world, according to LeGant.

There are beings that feed on sexual crime, on war, on negative thoughts, on control, on punishment, and on specific kinds of illness. "The more common beings in anxiety are 'punishment beings,' 'victim beings,' and 'hopelessness beings,'" he says, although the beings present depend entirely upon the individual.

LeGant knows about these beings through his "reading" of hundreds of people in the course of his work as a psychic healer. Over the years, he has repeatedly encountered these different types of beings in clients' energy fields.

The thoughts and emotions that people with anxiety disorder experience have a lot to do with the beings in their space. Whether we are aware of it or not, we all are telepathic, meaning we can pick up on others' thoughts. This telepathic wiring is the source of the transmittal of thoughts. For example, you might be excited about changing your life in some way, and then you get this foreign thought telling you, "You can't do this, you'll fail, it's not going to work, it's hopeless, it's useless." That is the being in your energy field *talking* to you. "If it's a really nasty being, like a 'suicide being,' it will say, 'It's so hopeless, you may as well kill yourself, that's what you need to do,' and then the person is in so much pain that that's what ends up happening," says LeGant. "Those thoughts can be very intense and quite overwhelming."

The problem is that most people don't realize that these are not their thoughts and they think that this is how they feel. People who are not developed clairvoyantly can't see the negative energy or distinguish its influence from their own emotions, so it is able to influence them and create confusion and angst. Influence by a being is often the case in people who go from doctor to doctor or other healer looking for a solution to their problem, to no avail. "What they need is someone to help them move the beings out of their energy field," which is what a spiritual healer such as LeGant does.

Pain Ridges and Core Pictures

In order to attach to people, the beings need something to anchor into. That something is pain, in the form of pain ridges and core pictures within people.

Pain ridges are energy blockages in the body that are formed during traumatic experiences. The pain associated with a trauma is stored in the body as a block of emotional energy, a pain ridge. "The beings plug into those pain ridges, into that old emotional energy, and it's like twisting a knife in someone's back," says LeGant. "They stimulate the old energies so the person continues to experience or sit in old emotion that has nothing to do with what's going on in present time."

Beings also attach to what are called "core pictures." These are made up of the emotions, thoughts, and sensory information associated with a trauma and are stored in the subconscious. Naturally, the content of core pictures is unique to each individual, but, as with the beings that are present, LeGant has seen common themes to the core pictures in clients with anxiety. In general, these pictures tend to be those of invalidation, punishment, and hopelessness. The core pictures provide another anchor for beings who feed on that type of energy. The beings then keep that energy strong, active, and "lit up," as LeGant refers to it—like a spotlight on a picture.

Death pictures are also commonly present in anxiety. "Some people have anxiety over groups of people and they may have death pictures from past lives where they were killed by mobs," notes LeGant.

Death pictures are also commonly present in anxiety. "Some people have anxiety over groups of people and they may have death pictures from past lives where they were killed by mobs," notes LeGant. "Most of the phobias are pretty easy to get rid of, whether it's fear of drowning or fear of heights. It's almost always a past-life picture of how they died, and the picture somehow got stimulated in this life."

For psychics, attuned as they are to nonphysical forces and the spirit realm, the existence of past lives is a working, empirical reality. For those who are not as in tune with their psychic abilities, the concept of past lives may arouse skepticism. It is not necessary to believe, however, in order to be healed psychically. Regardless of one's conceptual model, the healing will clear the energies and pictures that are contributing to a person's present anxiety state or interfering with their optimal functioning in other ways.

Death pictures contain the thoughts, emotions, and concepts of that long-ago moment of death. The body is always in present time, however, so it experiences the replaying of this pain as though it were happening *now*. "When the body gets stuck in a death picture, it will feel like it's dying," says LeGant. "It will experience what went on in that lifetime, and there's no rational explanation for where that emotion or that fear is coming from."

Again, prescription medications will numb people to the painful reenactment of their core pictures, but the pictures are still there.

Spiritual Healing

LeGant prefers to call what he does "spiritual healing" rather than "psychic healing," because the former is a more accurate description of what he is in fact doing, which is clearing the blockages to a person's connection to Spirit. He refers to this higher power as "the Supreme Being," which reflects its primacy over all the destructive beings that can occupy one's energy field. A strong connection to the Supreme Being is the best protection against the "negative beings," who cannot thrive in this atmosphere.

Spiritual healing involves erasing the core pictures, removing the pain ridges, and clearing all the negative beings from the person's energy field, says LeGant. Again, the content of all of this is unique to the individual, so the healing is never the same from one person to the next. In a session, LeGant and the client sit across from each other in comfortable chairs. To do his work, he goes into a light trance and, with eyes closed, "reads" what is happening in the client and sets about clearing the energy. Clients can choose to close their eyes or not during the process. By its very nature, psychic work does not require the client to be present. Spiritual healing can also be done over the phone, which is how LeGant and many of his colleagues work most of the time.

The first week after the first session is usually very intense, LeGant notes. He calls this a growth period, which is somewhat like the "healing crisis" well known to natural medicine practitioners. "The core pictures are like the keystone in an arch. When you pull the keystone out, a lot of stuff starts falling apart. Some people have built their life on their pain. You go in and take out that foundation and everything starts to go into flux; they redefine their reality. In the process of that, things die, and the person can feel like they're dying or like things are falling apart.

"After a week it starts to lighten up. After two weeks, you start to notice the joy underneath. It starts to come in and replace the pain with more lightness. If someone's in a crisis with their growth period, I just let them know that they can contact me. Usually they just need reassurance that it's normal. They don't need me to do anything."

In the case of anxiety, LeGant has found it easy to clear in most cases. Then, however, the client has to adjust to life without panic. "Panic attacks are very frightening to go through. It's not just fear. You can get dizzy, disoriented, lose your ability to hear and process, and just black out. Just the fear of having a panic attack can cause one." It is understandable that people would want to avoid the situations that brought on their panic before. In addition, "some people have been in it for so long that the thought of coming out of it is frightening to them," notes LeGant. It is familiar to them. "There's a level of safety there. They can stay home and not have to deal with certain things."

Some people become scared by feeling good after the energy that kept their anxiety in place is removed. Feeling good "lights up another layer of pictures for them." These might be from when they were children and the family subtly invalidated them when they were creative or having fun. This kind of invalidation is typically subconscious, not something that family members maliciously intend to do, says LeGant. A core picture forms around the belief that when they are feeling joyful or creating what they want, something bad is going to happen. The invalidation beings and the punishment beings attach to this type of core picture.

In these cases, the pictures and beings that make it uncomfortable for them to be happy and successful in their goals need to be removed. After being cleared, people are able to let in their success more and stop destroying it, but they need to move at their pace.

"They need to let one little thing materialize and realize they're n. going to die. They let another thing in, and they realize they're fine, that this is a good thing, no bomb's about to explode. They'll let in the next thing, and then they can start creating that success."

It is also necessary for people with anxiety to learn how to handle their sensitivity, so they will not go back to absorbing foreign energies, says LeGant. More specifically, his message is that you need to learn how to "be senior to energy" and how to define your own reality. This means not letting the beings or other people's energy determine your reality. In his Psychic School courses, LeGant teaches people how to accomplish this.

 There are many psychic healers, but not all work in the way described in this chapter. In addition to Leon LeGant (see appendix B: Resources for contact information for him and the Psychic School), graduates of the Berkeley Psychic Institute, of which LeGant is one, use some of these techniques (Berkeley Psychic Institute, Berkeley, CA; tel: 510-548-8020; website: www.berkeleypsychic.com). Lisa French, one of LeGant's teachers, also does psychic healings as described in this chapter and runs the Clairvoyant Center of Hawaii. For Lisa French, tel: 808-328-0747; website: www.magicisle.com. For the Clairvoyant Center, tel: 808-329-ROSE (7673); website: www.clairvoyanthawaii.org.

Joan: 20 Years of Panic

Joan, 45, suffered from severe panic attacks, for which she had been hospitalized in the past. She couldn't leave the house because being out in public brought on an attack. This meant she couldn't work and had no social life. This had been going on since she was in her mid-twenties. She had been on various antianxiety medications and had undergone a lot of individual and group therapy in an attempt to solve this debilitating problem. The drugs would numb her out, but she still couldn't leave the house.

In Joan's case, it took one session to clear her. There were a number of factors contributing to her panic, says LeGant. First, she was hypersensitive, which made her vulnerable to anxiety. Second, she had a number of death pictures from past lives. These death pictures were the major issue in clearing, rather than core pictures from her childhood. Third, as a spirit, this was the first time she had come into a body on this planet, so everything was new and overwhelming to her.

"Her past-life pictures were from other lifetimes on other planets, where she incarnated into alien environments and was attacked by mobs and killed," explains LeGant. As a result of her past-life pictures, Joan had a fear of being different and at the same time had always felt different from everyone else. This feeling kept the death pictures constantly stimulated. Her core belief was that if people saw who she really was, she'd get killed.

While many people may be tempted to dismiss the idea of lifetimes on other planets as ridiculous, the truth is that we don't know what other realities are informing who we are and how we feel in our present lives. When it comes down to it, science has no idea what causes mental problems such as panic attacks and other anxiety disorders. Yes, neurotransmitter imbalance is the current hypothesis, but that is not a causal explanation. What threw the neurotransmitters off in the first place? Given that the nervous system is electrical in nature, it makes sense that some kind of energy interference is at work. Our understanding of energy fields, as well as psychic phenomena, is so limited as yet that we have little basis for conclusions as to what may or may not be true. The beneficial results of Joan's psychic healing suggest that what LeGant did was a necessary intervention.

What LeGant understood when he "read" Joan was that her past-life pictures and the fear associated with them were interfering with her present life. "Any exposure out in public brought those fears up—fears that had no basis in this lifetime—and she could not function," explains LeGant. "She needed to be cleared of the death pictures. She needed a spirit-to-spirit validation that it's okay to be unique and also a 'hello' to who she is and what she is doing here in the body."

Joan came to LeGant again eight months after their first session to consult with him on an entirely different matter, a relationship issue. Relationships had been out of the question for her eight months before. Joan told him then that she had experienced no further panic attacks since their session, but she had needed to go through an adjustment period. It took her a few months to get used to being out in public and to trust that she wasn't going to have an attack. Once she was able to do that, she slowly began to restructure her life, taking little steps so she would be sure of herself. She got a job and started to create a social network, her panic now back in the past where it belonged.

Shamanic Healing

Shamanism is "perhaps the oldest form of practical spirituality in the world, originating in the time of Ice Age people, going back as far as 35,000 B.C."[186]

It is also practiced virtually everywhere in the world. A shaman is someone who has gone through advanced initiation into the "hidden" realm. The shaman uses the knowledge gained for healing and the good of the community. Despite the different label, shamanic healing is actually psychic healing. The terms are separated in this chapter to delineate indigenous shamanic practice from psychic healing that is not rooted in traditional ritual.

Malidoma Patrice Somé, Ph.D., is an internationally celebrated African shaman, diviner, and teacher who brings the healing wisdom of the Dagara tribe to the West. Dagara country is an area situated at the intersection of Ghana, the Ivory Coast, and Burkina Faso (formerly Upper Volta) in western Africa. Dr. Somé left his homeland to study in Europe and the United States and holds three master's degrees and two doctorates from the Sorbonne and Brandeis University. He has authored two books, *Ritual: Power, Healing, and Community* and *Of Water and the Spirit.*

The latter is his moving autobiography, which tells of his kidnap at the age of four by Jesuit missionaries who kept him prisoner and trained him as a missionary until at 20 he managed to escape. After an arduous trip back to his village, he underwent an initiation that restored him to his people and opened the way to

163

The Natural Medicine Guide to Anxiety

> ## In Their Own Words
>
> *"Suddenly, it was all clear to me. I wasn't going to die, I wasn't insane. Whatever was wrong with me, it sounded like here was finally someone who understood."*[187]
> —a woman with agoraphobia, upon seeing a television program on panic disorder

his shamanic practice. While conducting workshops and classes around the world, Dr. Somé maintains close connection with his village in Burkina Faso.

One of the things Dr. Somé encountered when he first came to the United States in 1980 for graduate study was how this country deals with mental illness. When a fellow student was sent to a mental institute due to "nervous depression," Dr. Somé went to visit him.

"I was so shocked. That was the first time I was brought face to face with what is done here to people exhibiting the same symptoms I've seen in my village." What struck Dr. Somé was that the attention given to such symptoms was based on pathology, on the idea that the condition is something that needs to stop. This was in complete opposition to the way his culture views such a situation. As he looked around the stark ward at the patients, some in straitjackets, some zoned out on medications, others screaming, he observed to himself, "So this is how the healers who are attempting to be born are treated in this culture. What a loss! What a loss that a person who is finally being aligned with a power from the other world is just being wasted."

On the ward, Dr. Somé also saw a lot of "beings" hanging around the patients, "entities" that are invisible to most people but that shamans and some psychics are able to see. "They were causing the crisis in these people," he says. It appeared to him that these beings were trying to get the medications and their effects out of the bodies of the people the beings were trying to merge with, and were increasing the patients' pain in the process.

"The beings were acting almost like some kind of excavator in the energy field of the people. They were really fierce about that. The people they were doing that to were just screaming and yelling." Dr. Somé couldn't stay in that environment and had to leave.

This approach to mental illness was diametrically opposed to how such illness is treated in Dr. Somé's culture. Mental disorders are spiritual emergencies, spiritual crises, and need to be regarded as such, he says. The Dagara people view these crises as "good news from the other world." The person going through the crisis has been chosen as a medium for a message to the community that needs to be communicated from the spirit realm. The community helps the person reconcile the energies of both worlds—"the world of the spirit that he or she is merged with, and the village and community."

That person is able then to serve as a bridge between the worlds and help the living with information and healing they need. Thus, the spiritual crisis ends with the birth of another healer. "The other world's relationship with our world is one of sponsorship," Dr. Somé explains. "More often than not, the knowledge and skills that arise from this kind of merger are a knowledge or a skill that is provided directly from the other world."

The "beings" or "spirits" who were increasing the pain of the inmates on the mental hospital ward were actually attempting to merge with the inmates in order to get messages through to this world. The people they had chosen to merge with were getting no assistance in learning how to be a bridge between the worlds, and the beings' attempts to merge were thwarted. The result was the sustaining of the initial disorder of energy and the aborting of the birth of a healer.

"The Western culture has consistently ignored the birth of the healer," states Dr. Somé. "Consequently, there will be a tendency from the other world to keep trying as many people as possible in an attempt to get somebody's attention. They have to try harder." The spirits are drawn to people whose senses have not been anesthetized. "The sensitivity is pretty much read as an invitation to come in," he notes.

Those who develop so-called mental disorders are those who are sensitive, which is viewed in Western culture as oversensitivity. Indigenous cultures don't see it that way, and, as a result, sensitive people don't experience themselves as overly sensitive. In the West, "it is the overload of the culture they're in that is just wrecking them," observes Dr. Somé. The frenetic pace, the bombardment of the senses, and the violent energy that characterize Western culture can overwhelm sensitive people.

Anxiety and Purpose

With anxiety and depression, which are virtual epidemics in the United States, Dr. Somé has found that the main underlying problem is disconnection from one's life purpose. This disconnection "leaves room for foreign energies to come in that don't have anything to do with the kind of promise the person made before coming into this world," the promise of what one will fulfill in one's life. "When you make a promise like that, and you come here and you start doing something else, you're subject to anxiety and depression."

The shaman can see what a person's purpose is. "The divination doesn't hide these kinds of things," says Dr. Somé. The shaman's task in this case is to tell people their purpose, but only after preparing them through ritual so they are in a position to understand what is revealed. The ritual used is called a "dupulo" and works to correct the changes done to the original promise. "It's like a disruption of the current path the person is in. It prepares the space for the promise to come alive in the person." After the ritual, the shaman lets a week or two pass, to let it sink in, and then helps the person to become consciously aware of their promise, the specifics of their purpose.

At that point, it is up to them to "take it or leave it," Dr. Somé says. "If they decide to not fulfill that purpose, they'll find themselves back in anxiety or depression." The choice is theirs—they can choose to be anxious or depressed or choose to be aligned with their path.

Dr. Somé gives the example of a man whose promise before being born, the reason why he came into this world, was to work at providing homes for people. "That's a metaphor for a variety of things. One is the actual physical home, another is helping people to feel comfortable with themselves. The man shows up here, finds out how difficult it is, and winds up working in a factory." After receiving the information about his purpose, "he can either start looking into the possibility of being a home-builder or a healer who brings stability or groundedness to other people, or not."

Longing for Connection

Another common thread that Dr. Somé has noticed in anxiety and depression is "a very ancient ancestral energy that has been placed in stasis, that finally is coming out in the person." His job then is to trace it back, to go back in time to discover what that spirit is. In most cases, the spirit is connected to nature, especially with mountains or big rivers, he says.

In the case of mountains, as an example to explain the phenomenon, "it's a spirit of the mountain that is walking side by side with the person and, as a result, creating a time-space distortion that is affecting the person caught in it." What is needed is a merger or alignment of the two energies, "so the person and the mountain spirit become one." Again, the shaman conducts a specific ritual to bring about this alignment.

Dr. Somé believes that he encounters this situation so often in the United States because "most of the fabric of this country is made up of the energy of the machine, and

Another common thread that Dr. Somé has noticed in anxiety and depression is "a very ancient ancestral energy that has been placed in stasis, that finally is coming out in the person." His job then is to trace it back, to go back in time to discover what that spirit is.

the result of that is the disconnection and the severing of the past. You can run from the past, but you can't hide from it." The ancestral spirit of the natural world comes visiting. "It's not so much what the spirit wants as it is what the person wants," he says. "The spirit sees in us a call for something grand, something that will make life meaningful, and so the spirit is responding to that."

That call, which we don't even know we are making, reflects "a strong longing for a profound connection, a connection that transcends materialism and possession of things and moves into a tangible cosmic dimension. Most of this longing is unconscious, but for spirits, conscious or unconscious doesn't make any difference." They respond to either.

As part of the ritual to merge the mountain and human energy, those who are receiving the "mountain energy" are sent to a mountain area of their choice, where they pick up a stone that calls to them. They bring that stone back for the rest of the ritual and then keep it as a companion; some even carry it around with them. "The presence of the stone does a lot in tuning the perceptive ability of the person," notes Dr. Somé. "They receive all kinds of information that they can make use of, so it's like they get some tangible guidance from the other world as to how to live their life."

When it is the "river energy," those being called go to the river and, after speaking to the river spirit, find a water stone to bring back for the same kind of ritual as with the mountain spirit.

"People think something extraordinary must be done in an extraordinary situation like this," he says. That's not usually the case. Sometimes it is as simple as carrying a stone.

Rituals for the West

One of the gifts a shaman can bring to the Western world is to help people rediscover ritual, which is so sadly lacking. "The abandonment of ritual can be devastating. From the spiritual viewpoint, ritual is inevitable and necessary if one is to live," Dr. Somé writes in *Ritual: Power, Healing, and Community.* "To say that ritual is needed in the industrialized world is an understatement. We have seen in my own people that it is probably impossible to live a sane life without it."[188]

Dr. Somé did not feel that the rituals from his traditional village could be transferred as is to the West, so over his years of shamanic work here, he has designed rituals that meet the very different needs of this culture. Although the rituals change according to the individual or the group involved, he finds that there is a need for certain rituals in general.

One of these involves helping people discover that their distress is coming from the fact that they are "called by beings from the other world to cooperate with them in doing healing work." Ritual allows them to move out of the distress and accept that calling.

Another ritual need relates to initiation. In indigenous cultures all over the world, young people are initiated into adulthood when they reach a certain age. The lack of such initiation in the West is part of the crisis that people are in here, says Dr. Somé. He urges communities to bring together "the creative juices of people who have had this kind of experience, in an attempt to come up with some kind of an alternative ritual that would at least begin to put a dent in this kind of crisis."

Another ritual that repeatedly speaks to the needs of those coming to him for help entails making a bonfire and then putting into the bonfire "items that are symbolic of issues carried inside the individuals. . . . It might be the issues of anger and frustration against an ancestor who has left a legacy of murder and enslavement—or anything, things that the descendant has to live with," he explains. "If these are approached as things that are blocking the human imagination, the person's life purpose, and even the person's view of life as something that can improve, then it makes sense to begin thinking in terms of how to turn that blockage into a roadway that can lead to something more creative and more fulfilling."

The example of issues with an ancestor touches on rituals designed by Dr. Somé that address a serious dysfunction in Western society, and in the process "trigger enlightenment" in participants. These are ancestral rituals, and the dysfunction they are aimed at is the mass turning-of-the-back on ancestors. Some of the spirits trying to come through, as described earlier, may be "ancestors who want to merge with a descendant in an attempt to heal what they weren't able to do while in their physical body."

"Unless the relationship between the living and the dead is in balance, chaos ensues," he says. "The Dagara believe that, if such an imbalance exists, it is the duty of the living to heal their ancestors. If these ancestors are not healed, their sick energy will haunt the souls and psyches of those who are responsible for helping them."[189]

The rituals focus on healing the relationship with our ancestors, both specific issues of an individual ancestor and the larger cultural issues contained in our past. Dr. Somé has seen extraordinary healing occur at these rituals.

Taking a sacred ritual approach to anxiety, depression, and other disturbances rather than regarding the person as a pathological case gives the person affected—and indeed the community at large—the opportunity to begin looking at it from that vantage point too, which leads to "a whole plethora of opportunities and ritual initiative that can be very, very beneficial to everyone present," states Dr. Somé.

Healing and Belonging

With shamanic healing, as with any other kind of healing, there needs to be an agreement with the recipient that they are indeed willing to heal. "There's a lot of resistance to healing," comments Dr. Somé. "There's more of an acceptance of the pathology as a means of getting attention than there is a desire to get out of there." He cites the societal isolationism or tendency to be alone in your own space as one of the contributing factors to this pattern. Illness is one path to a sense of belonging.

"We have to understand that there is in the human being a certain instinct towards belonging. When that doesn't happen, the creative self goes to heavy-duty work to try to figure out all kinds of different ways to belong. Pathology can become a very cozy area of belonging, and people will hang onto their own pain because that's what makes them feel alive."

Dr. Somé helps open people's eyes to another kind of belonging. It doesn't happen overnight, but there is "a gradual emergence in the person of a certain perception of themselves and of the world that makes them gradually realize that they do fit, that in fact, the way they used to feel has shifted from a pathology to a healership." They see that they actually have a gift that can benefit people.

With this realization, they enter a completely different arena of belonging. They are now part of the group that has something to give to the world. "Giving is a very tangible form of belonging," says Dr. Somé. This approach is a powerful way of turning anxiety and depression around. "The reorientation of the person away from isolation into a sense of collective belonging transcends dramatically the feeling of being useless."

With foreign energies removed by shamanic or psychic healing, and a sense of purpose and belonging restored, the individual can move from anxiety to balance in body, mind, and spirit.

Afterword

Many of our lives are ruled by fear. Rather than acting based on what we truly want to do, we often act out of fear. Fear prevents us from realizing our dreams. It suppresses creativity, strangles joy, stops love from growing, and keeps people apart. Fear prevents members of different cultures from recognizing each other's humanity. Fear starts wars. Individual lives and the whole planet are suffering from this reign of fear.

In this context, anxiety is not only a personal issue, but has repercussions that extend beyond the individual, especially given the epidemic proportions anxiety has reached in our world today. Anxiety is preventing too many people from living to their full potential. That loss affects us all. The message here is that you are not alone, either in your anxiety or in the losses you suffer when anxiety runs your life.

The message of this book is that you don't have to live with crippling anxiety. And you don't have to resign yourself simply to coping with your "disability." By systematically addressing your particular cluster of imbalances—in body, mind, and spirit—you can find your way out of anxiety and begin to live the life you were meant to live.

When anxiety becomes a permanent presence or interferes with living, it is a signal that something is wrong. The body has its own wisdom, and a panic attack can be seen as a wake-up call, alerting you that something needs your attention. By heeding the call and seeking to identify and correct what is amiss in body, mind, and spirit, you not only alleviate your anxiety, but also benefit all aspects of your health.

As you learned in this book, the imbalances that can contribute to an anxiety disorder range from nutritional deficiencies and allergies to energy disturbances and psychospiritual issues. This book has shown you practical ways to reverse these factors. The imbalances underlying your anxiety can produce many other mental and physical symptoms and health problems as well. Restoring balance on all levels is thus both an antianxiety measure and good preventive medicine.

The restoration of balance does not mean that you will never feel fearful again. Fear is a natural part of life, and certainly there is much to be anxious about in the world today. But it is possible to move forward with our lives despite the transient anxiety we may feel. Restoring balance gives your body, mind, and spirit the strength they need to meet the fears and anxieties of life and not be ruled by them. In releasing yourself from the reign of fear, you benefit you and everyone in your life and contribute to stopping the escalating epidemic of anxiety.

Appendix A
Professional Degrees and Titles

C.M.P.	Certified Massage Practitioner
L.Ac.	Licensed Acupuncturist
L.C.S.W.	Licensed Clinical Social Worker
N.M.D.	Doctor of Naturopathic Medicine
N.D.	Doctor of Naturopathy
O.M.D.	Oriental Medical Doctor
R.M.T.	Registered Massage Therapist

Appendix B
Resources

Practitioners in This Book

Ira J. Golchehreh, L.Ac., O.M.D.
2175-D Francisco Blvd.
San Rafael, CA 94901
Tel: 415-484-4411

Licensed as an acupuncturist, doctor of oriental medicine, doctor of alternative medicine, and qualified medical evaluator (Q.M.E.) for the State of California, Dr. Golchehreh runs a general practice specializing in internal and external disorders, pain-related disorders, and sports/orthopedic medicine.

Patricia Kaminski
Flower Essence Society
P.O. Box 459
Nevada City, CA 95959
Tel: 800-736-9222 (U.S. and Canada) or 530-265-9163
Fax: 530-265-0584
E-mail: pkaminski@flowersociety.org
Website: www.flowersociety.org

Patricia Kaminski is an herbalist, flower essence therapist, co-director of the Flower Essence Society, author of *Flowers That Heal*, and coauthor of *Flower Essence Repertory*.

The Flower Essence Society is an international membership organization of health practitioners, researchers, students, and others interested in deepening their knowledge of flower essence therapy. FES is devoted to research and education, and offers training and certification programs, and publications. The Society also provides a free networking service for finding a practitioner in your area.

Kendra Barnett, whose case history appears in chapter 6, is a flower essence practitioner who trained with Patricia Kaminski and the Flower Essence Society. She runs a private practice and also works for the society. She can be reached at P.O. Box 1053, Nevada City, CA 95959; e-mail kendra@fesflowers.com.

Dietrich Klinghardt, M.D., Ph.D.
1200 112th Ave. NE, Ste. A100
Bellevue, WA 98004
Tel: 425-688-8818

Dr. Klinghardt specializes in Neural Therapy, Applied Psychoneurobiology, and Family Systems Therapy, which addresses the transgenerational energy legacies at the root of illness.

Carola M. Lage-Roy, Naturopath-Homoeopath
(Heilpraktikerin Homoeopathie)
2421 Summerhill Dr.
Encinitas, CA 92024
Tel: 760-943-7697 or 760-943-8885
In Germany:
Breite 2
82418 Murnau, Germany
Tel: 49-8841-4455
Fax: 49-8841-4298
E-mail: homoeopathy@ravi-roy.de (note the European spelling of
    homoeopathy)
Website: www.ravi-roy.de

In addition to their homoeopathic practice, Lage-Roy and her husband, Ravi Roy, run Lage & Roy Publishing Company and have written 28 books on homoeopathy, including *Homoeopathic Guide: Vaccination Damage, Homoeopathic Guide: Infectious Diseases of Children, The Homoeopathic Family Home-Care,* and *Bioweapons and Homoeopathy.*

They also run the Ravi Roy Teaching and Research Institute for Homoeopathy and offer a correspondence course in homoeopathy.

Rev. Leon S. LeGant
The Psychic School
Tel: 800-951-8042
E-mail: leon@psychicschool.com
Website: www.psychicschool.com

LeGant is a psychic clairvoyant, spiritual healer, and executive director of the Psychic School, a nonprofit organization dedicated to the development of psychic abilities, spiritual awareness, and self-healing. The School offers readings, classes, retreats, short- and long-term training programs, and long-distance spiritual education.

Thomas M. Rau, M.D.
Paracelsus Klinik Lustmühle
CH-9062 Lustmühle b. St. Gallen
Switzerland
Tel: 41-71-335-71-71
Fax: 41-71-335-71-00
E-mail: dr.thomas.rau@paracelsus.ch
Website: www.paracelsus.ch

The Paracelsus Klinik is a center for European biological medicine and holistic dentistry. All chronic diseases are treated in this clinic, where medical doctors and dentists work together under one roof.

Judyth Reichenberg-Ullman, N.D., L.C.S.W.
The Northwest Center for Homeopathic Medicine
131 Third Ave. N.
Edmonds, WA 98020

Tel: 425-774-5599

Website: www.healthyhomeopathy.com

In practice with her husband, Robert Ullman, Dr. Reichenberg-Ullman is a licensed naturopathic physician board certified in homeopathy. She has been practicing for 18 years and is the author/coauthor of six books on homeopathic medicine, including *Prozac Free, Ritalin-Free Kids,* and *Whole Woman Homeopathy.*

Tony Roffers, Ph.D.

3542 Fruitvale Ave., #218

Oakland, CA 94602-2327

Tel: 510-531-6730

E-mail: tonyroffers@earthlink.net

Dr. Roffers is a licensed psychologist whose private practice with adult clients emphasizes Thought Field Therapy and Seemorg Matrix Work for a wide variety of problems including anxiety, panic disorder, PTSD, depression, addiction, and food and inhalant sensitivities.

Malidoma Patrice Somé, Ph.D.

236 West East Ave., Ste. A, PMB 199

Chico, CA 95926

Tel: 530-894-0740

E-mail: rowenap@jps.net (Rowena Pantaleon, Dr. Somé's assistant)

Website: www.malidoma.com

Dr. Somé is an African shaman, diviner, and teacher who brings the healing wisdom of the Dagara tribe to the West.

Zannah Steiner, C.M.P., R.M.T.

Soma Therapy Centre

2607 W. 16th Ave.

Vancouver, BC V6K 3C2

Canada

Tel: 604-731-7883

E-mail: soma@intouch.bc.ca

Website: www.somatherapy.info

The Centre offers a range of soma (body) therapies, particularly utilizing CranioSacral Therapy, Visceral Manipulation, and SomatoEmotional Release to address the root causes of a disorder. Other therapies include acupuncture, chiropractic, psychological counseling, massage, and hydrotherapy. Among the conditions commonly treated are anxiety, depression, addictions, chronic fatigue, immune deficiencies, chronic pain, paralysis, autism, developmental delays, and ADD.

Endnotes

Introduction

1. Jean M. Twenge, "The Age of Anxiety? Birth Cohort Change in Anxiety and Neuroticism, 1952–1993," *Journal of Personality and Social Psychology* 79:6 (December 2000): 1007–21; available on the Internet at www.apa.org/journals/psp/psp7961007.html#c25s. NAMI, "Anxiety Disorders," available on the Internet at the NAMI Website: www.nami.org; or contact NAMI (National Alliance for the Mentally Ill), Colonial Place Three, 2107 Wilson Blvd., Suite 300, Alexandria, VA 22201-3042; tel: 888-999-NAMI (6264) or 703-524-7600.

2. Mary Ellin Lerner, "Facing Your Fear," *USA Weekend* (September 29–October 1, 2000): 8-9. Michele Meyer, "There's Help for Social Phobia," *Parade Magazine* (December 17, 2000): 10.

3. NAMI, "Anxiety Disorders."

4. Freedom From Fear, "Anxiety Disorders," available on the Internet at www.freedomfromfear.org/aanx_factsheet.asp?id=17; or contact Freedom From Fear, 308 Seaview Ave., Staten Island, NY 10305; tel: 718-351-1717.

5. C. J. L. Murray and A. D. Lopez, eds., *Summary: The Global Burden of Disease: A Comprehensive Assessment of Mortality and Disability from Diseases, Injuries, and Risk Factors in 1990 and Projected to 2020* (Cambridge, MA: Harvard School of Public Health on Behalf of the World Health Organization and the World Bank, Harvard University Press, 1996). Available on the Internet at:

www.who.int/msa/mnh/ems/dalys/intro.htm. Cited in U.S. Department of Health and Human Services, "Mental Health: A Report of the Surgeon General, Executive Summary," (Rockville, MD: U.S. Department of Health and Human Services, Substance Abuse and Mental Health Services Administration, Center for Mental Health Services, National Institutes of Health, National Institute of Mental Health, 1999): ix.

6. C. J. L. Murray and A. D. Lopez, eds., *Summary.*

7. R. C. Kessler et al., "A Methodology for Estimating the 12-Month Prevalence of Serious Mental Illness," in: R. W. Manderscheid and M. J. Henderson, eds., *Mental Health, United States, 1999* (Rockville, MD: Center for Mental Health Services, 1998): 99–109.

8. Center for Mental Health Services, *Survey of Mental Health Organizations and General Mental Health Services* (Rockville, MD: Center for Mental Health Services, 1998).

9. 1990 is the most recent year for which estimates are available, according to "Mental Health: A Report of the U.S. Surgeon General" (Rockville, MD: U.S. Department of Health and Human Services, Substance Abuse and Mental Health Services Administration, Center for Mental Health Services, National Institutes of Health, National Institute of Mental Health, 1999). D. P. Rice and L. S. Miller, "The Economic Burden of Schizophrenia: Conceptual and Methodological Issues, and Cost Estimates," in M. Moscarelli, A. Rupp, and N. Sartorious, eds., *Handbook of Mental Health Economics and Health Policy: Schizophrenia,* vol. 1 (New York: John Wiley and Sons, 1996): 321–4.

10. The full text of the letter is available on the Internet at: www.moshersoteria.com

1: What Is Anxiety and Who Suffers from It?

11. NIMH, "Anxiety Disorders," National Institute of Mental Health (NIH Publication No. 00-3879, reprinted 2000); available on the Internet at: www.nimh.nih.gov/anxiety/anxiety.cfm.

12. Jerilyn Ross, *Triumph Over Fear: A Book of Help and Hope for People with Anxiety, Panic Attacks, and Phobias* (New York: Bantam Books, 1994): 73.

13. Freedom From Fear, "Misdiagnosis of Anxiety Disorders

Costs U.S. Billions Abstract," available from Freedom From Fear, 308 Seaview Ave., Staten Island, NY 10305; tel: 718-351-1717; Website: www.freedomfromfear.org.

14. National Alliance for the Mentally Ill (NAMI), "Anxiety Disorders," available on the Internet at: www.nami.org; or contact NAMI, Colonial Place Three, 2107 Wilson Blvd., Suite 300, Alexandria, VA 22201-3042; tel: (888) 999-NAMI (6264) or (703) 524-7600.

15. Anxiety Disorders Association of America (ADAA), "Statistics and Facts About Anxiety Disorders"; available on the Internet at www.adaa.org/mediaroom/index.cfm or contact ADAA, 8730 Georgia Ave., Ste. 600, Silver Spring, MD 20910; tel: 240-485-1001.

16. Ibid.

17. Jerilyn Ross, *Triumph Over Fear,* xv.

18. American Psychiatric Association, *DSM-IV-TR* (*Diagnostic and Statistical Manual of Mental Disorders, 4th Edition, Text Revision*) (Washington, DC: American Psychiatric Association, 2000): 432.

19. Harold H. Bloomfield, M.D., *Healing Anxiety Naturally* (New York: Perennial Press, 1999): 5.

20. *DSM-IV-TR,* 433–4.

21. L. N. Robins and D. A. Regier, eds., *Psychiatric Disorders in America: The Epidemiologic Catchment Area Study* (New York: Free Press, 1991).

22. Jerilyn Ross, *Triumph Over Fear,* xiv.

23. *DSM-IV-TR,* 435–6.

24. *DSM-IV-TR,* 443, 449.

25. *DSM-IV-TR,* 445.

26. *DSM-IV-TR,* 445–7.

27. P. L. Amies, M. G. Gelder, and P. M. Shaw, "Social Phobia: A Comparative Clinical Study," *British Journal of Psychiatry* 142 (1983): 174–9.

28. Shirley Babior and Carol Goldman, *Overcoming Panic, Anxiety, & Phobias: New Strategies to Free Yourself from Worry and Fear* (Duluth, MN: Whole Person Associates, 1996): 71–2.

29. *DSM-IV-TR,* 456.

30. John R. Marshall, M.D., and Suzanne Lipsett, *Social Phobia: From Shyness to Stage Fright* (New York: Basic Books, 1994): 152.

31. *DSM-IV-TR,* 452–3.

32. *DSM-IV-TR,* 476.

33. NIMH, "Anxiety Disorders."

34. *DSM-IV-TR,* 473–4.

35. *Taber's Cyclopedic Medical Dictionary,* 17th ed. (Philadelphia, PA: F. A. Davis Company, 1993): 2040.

36. *DSM-IV-TR,* 458–60.

37. NIMH, "Anxiety Disorders."

38. *DSM-IV-TR,* 466.

39. *DSM-IV-TR,* 465–6.

40. Jerilyn Ross, *Triumph Over Fear,* xvi.

41. NAMI, "Anxiety Disorders."

42. Jerilyn Ross, *Triumph Over Fear,* 258.

43. R. Reid Wilson, Ph.D., *Don't Panic: Taking Control of Anxiety Attacks* (New York: Perennial Press, 1996): 98.

44. Muriel MacFarlane, R.N., M.A., *The Panic Attack, Anxiety, and Phobia Solutions Handbook* (Leucadia, CA: United Research Publishers, 1995): 192.

45. M. M. Weissman, "The Hidden Patient: Unrecognized Panic Disorder," *Journal of Clinical Psychiatry* 5: suppl. 11 (1990): 5–8. Cited in: Jonathan R. T. Davidson, M.D., "The Economic and Social Costs of Panic Disorder," article available on the Internet at: www.mmhc.com.

46. J. P. Lepine, J. M. Chignon, and M. Teherani, "Suicide Attempts in Patients with Panic Disorder," *Archives of General Psychiatry* 50:2 (1993): 144–9. Cited in: Frank J. Ayd, Jr., M.D., and Claudia Daileader, "The Correlation Between Suicide and Panic Disorder," *Psychiatric Times* 17:9 (September 2000); available on the Internet at: www.lorenbennett.org.

47. Ibid.

48. Rita Elkins, *Depression and Natural Medicine: A Nutritional Approach to Depression and Mood Swings* (Pleasant Grove, UT: Woodland Publishing, 1995): 16. Demitri Papolos, M.D., and Janice Papolos, *Overcoming Depression: The Definitive Resource for Patients and Families Who Live with Depression and Manic-Depression* (New York: HarperPerennial, 1997): 270.

49. Harold H. Bloomfield, *Healing Anxiety Naturally,* xii.

50. Douglas Hunt, M.D., and Len Mervyn, *No More Fears: The Nutritional Plan to Beat Anxiety* (New York: Warner, 1988).

51. "A Brief History of Anxiety Disorders," available on the Internet at: dubinserver.colorado.edu/prj/kng/history.html.

52. Demitri Papolos, M.D., and Janice Papolos, *Overcoming Depression: The Definitive Resource for Patients and Families Who Live with Depression and Manic-Depression*: 32–3.

53. Edward Shorter, *A History of Psychiatry: From the Era of the Asylum to the Age of Prozac* (New York: John Wiley and Sons, 1998).

54. Ibid.

55. Arthur Anderson, ed., "Anxiety-Panic History: Anxiety, Disorders and Treatments Throughout the Ages," available on the Internet at: http://anxiety-panic.com/history/h-main.htm.

56. Mary Ellin Lerner, "Facing Your Fear," *USA Weekend* (September 29–October 1, 2000): 8–9. Michele Meyer, "There's Help for Social Phobia," *Parade Magazine* (December 17, 2000): 10.

www.healthyplace.com/communities/anxiety/paems/people/.

www.algy.com/anxiety/famous.html.

www.ruhsagligi.org/pandost/english/famous_people_with_panic_attacks.htm.

www.geocities.com/spiroll2/celebs.html.

57. Jeffrey Kluger, "Fear Not! Phobias," *Time* (April 2, 2001): 61.

58. Arthur Anderson, "Anxiety-Panic History."

59. NIMH press release: "Anxiety Disorders Treatment Target: Amygdala Circuitry" (December 15, 1998), article on the Internet (www.nimh.nih.gov/events/pranxst.cfm); also released by the Anxiety Disorders Association of America (www.adaa.org). Harold H. Bloomfield, *Healing Anxiety Naturally*, 32.

60. S. L. Rauch and C. R. Savage, "Neuroimaging and Neuropsychology of the Striatum: Bridging Basic Science and Clinical Practice," *Psychiatric Clinics of North America* 20:4 (1997): 741–68. Daniel G. Amen, M.D., *Change Your Brain, Change Your Life* (New York: Three Rivers Press, 1998): 82.

61. E. C. Azmitia and P. M. Whitaker-Azmitia, "Awakening the Sleeping Giant: Anatomy and Plasticity of the Brain Serotonergic System," *Journal of Clinical Psychiatry* 52:12 suppl. (1991): 4–16. Cited in Joseph Glenmullen, M.D., *Prozac Backlash* (New York: Touchstone/Simon & Schuster, 2000): 16.

62. Julia Ross, M.A., *The Diet Cure* (New York: Penguin, 1999): 121.

63. Joseph Glenmullen, *Prozac Backlash*, 340.

64. *Taber's Cyclopedic Medical Dictionary*, 662, 1318.

65. Russell Jaffe, M.D., Ph.D., and Oscar Rogers Kruesi, M.D., "The Biochemical-Immunology Window: A Molecular View of Psychiatric Case Management," *Journal of Applied Nutrition* 44:2 (1992).

66. Eve Edelman, *Natural Healing for Schizophrenia and Other Common Mental Disorders*, 3rd ed. (Eugene, OR: Borage Books, 2001): 144.

67. Julia Ross, *The Diet Cure*, 120.

68. Joseph Glenmullen, *Prozac Backlash*, 16.

69. Peter R. Breggin, M.D., and David Cohen, Ph.D., *Your Drug May Be Your Problem: How and Why to Stop Taking Psychiatric Medications* (Reading, MA: Perseus Books, 1999): 71.

70. Ibid., 72.

71. Ibid., 71.

72. Raeann Dumont, *The Sky Is Falling: Understanding and Coping with Phobias, Panic, and Obsessive-Compulsive Disorders* (New York: W.W. Norton, 1996): 282.

73. Michael T. Murray, N.D., *Natural Alternatives to Prozac* (New York: Quill/William Morrow, 1996): 4.

74. Ibid.

75. Maryann Napoli, "A New Assessment of Depression Drugs," *HealthFacts* 24:7 (July 31, 1999): 4.

76. Joseph Glenmullen, *Prozac Backlash*, 299.

77. A. C. Pande and M. E. Sayler, "Adverse Events and Treatment Discontinuations in Fluoxetine Clinical Trials," *International Journal of Psychopharmacology* 8 (1993): 267–9.

78. Ronald Hoffman, "Beyond Prozac: Natural Therapies for Anxiety and Depression," *Innovation: The Health Letter of FAIM* (January 31, 1999): 10–11, 13, 15, 17, 19.

79. Breggin and Cohen, *Your Drug May Be Your Problem*, 55. Joseph Glenmullen, *Prozac Backlash*, 152–3.

80. Joseph Glenmullen, *Prozac Backlash*. Breggin and Cohen, *Your Drug May Be Your Problem*, 46–7.

2: Causes, Triggers, and Contributors

81. Richard Leviton, *The Healthy Living Space* (Charlottesville, VA: Hampton Roads, 2001): 2.

82. Ibid., 3.

83. "Doctors Warn Developmental Disabilities Epidemic from Toxins," *LDA (Learning Disabilities Association of America) Newsbriefs* 35:4 (July/August 2000): 3–5. Executive Summary from the Report by the Greater Boston Physicians for Social Responsibility, *In Harm's Way: Toxic Threats to Child Development,* available at www.igc.org/psr/ihw.htm.

84. Philip J. Landrigan, *Environmental Neurotoxicology,* (Washington, DC: National Academy Press, 1992): 2; cited in Richard Leviton, *The Healthy Living Space,* 13.

85. *DSM-IV-TR,* 430.

86. National Institute for Occupational Safety and Health, "Nonfatal Illness: Anxiety, Stress, and Neurotic Disorders," in *Worker Health Chartbook, 2000* (Washington, D.C.: NIOSH, 2000); available on the Internet at: www.cdc.gov/niosh/pdfs/2000-127o.pdf.

87. Reuters Health, "Chemical Sensitivity Tied to Anxiety, Depression" (2003); article on the Internet (http://12.42.224.153/HealthNews/Reuters/NewsStory1023200214.htm), reporting on article in *Journal of Occupational and Environmental Medicine* 44 (2002): 890–901.

88. G. E. Simon, "Psychiatric Symptoms in Multiple Chemical Sensitivity," *Toxicology and Industrial Health* 10:4–5 (1994): 487–96.

89. Sherry A. Rogers, M.D., *Depression: Cured at Last!* (Sarasota, FL: SK Publishing, 1997): 94.

90. John Foster, M.D., "Is Depression Natural in an Unnatural World?" *Well-Being Journal* (Spring 2001): 11; website: www.wellbeingjournal.com.

91. Dietrich Klinghardt, M.D., Ph.D., "Amalgam/Mercury Detox as a Treatment for Chronic Viral, Bacterial, and Fungal Illnesses," lecture presented at the Annual Meeting of the International and American Academy of Clinical Nutrition, San Diego, CA, September 1996.

92. Morton Walker, D.P.M., *Elements of Danger: Protect Yourself Against the Hazards of Modern Dentistry* (Charlottesville, VA: Hampton Roads, 2000): 138, 141.

93. Ronald J. Diamond, M.D., "Psychiatric Presentations of

Medical Illness: An Introduction for Non-Medical Mental Health Professionals," article on the Internet, revised January 7, 2002, available at www.alternativementalhealth.com/articles/diamond.htm. Dr. Larry Wilson, "Nutritional Causes of Anxiety and Panic Attacks," *ENcourage Newsletter* (1995), available on the ENcourage website: www.encourageconnection.com/art01.html.

94. Syd Baumel, *Dealing with Depression Naturally* (Los Angeles: Keats Publishing, 2000): 34.

95. Allan Sachs, D.C., C.C.N., *The Authoritative Guide to Grapefruit Seed Extract* (Mendocino, CA: LifeRhythm, 1997): 58.

96. Sherry Rogers, *Depression,* 165–7.

97. Ibid., 166.

98. Personal communication, 2001.

99. Carla Wills-Brandon, Ph.D., *Natural Mental Health: How to Take Control of Your Own Emotional Well-Being* (Carlsbad, CA: Hay House, 2000): 118.

100. Sherry Rogers, *Depression,* 460.

101. Ibid., 461–2.

102. Jerilyn Ross, *Triumph Over Fear: A Book of Help and Hope for People with Anxiety, Panic Attacks, and Phobias* (New York: Bantam Books, 1994): 257.

103. Michael T. Murray, N.D., and Joseph Pizzorno, N.D., *Encyclopedia of Natural Medicine* (Rocklin, CA: Prima Publishing, 1991): 395.

104. Harold H. Bloomfield, M.D., *Healing Anxiety Naturally* (New York: HarperPerennial, 1998): 52.

105. John N. Hathcock, *Nutritional Toxicology,* vol.1 (New York: Academic Press, 1982): 462. L. D. Steglink and L. J. Filer, Jr., eds., *Aspartame* (New York: Marcel Dekker, 1984): 350, 359. Bryan Ballantyne, Timothy Marrs, and Paul Turner, eds., *General and Applied Toxicology,* vol. 1 (New York: Stockton Press, 1993): 482.

106. "Aspartame Danger: Toxicity Effects of Aspartame Use," article on the Internet, available at: www.anxietypanic.com/aspartame.html. "Common Reactions," on the NOMSG web site: www.nomsg.com/reactions.html.

107. Leon Chaitow, *Thorson's Guide to Amino Acids* (London: Thorson, 1991): 95.

108. Susan C. Smolinske, *Handbook of Food, Drug, and Cosmetic Excipients* (Boca Raton, FL: CRC Press, 1992): 236.

109. Bernard Rimland, Ph.D., "The Feingold Diet: An Assessment of the Reviews by Marttes, by Kavale and Forness and Others," *Journal of Learning Disabilities* 16:6 (June/July 1983): 331. (Available from the Autism Research Institute, Publication #51.)

110. William Walsh, Ph.D., "The Critical Role of Nutrients in Severe Mental Symptoms," article available on the Internet (www.alternativementalhealth.com/articles/article-pffeiffer.htm).

111. Ibid.

112. Eva Edelman, *Natural Healing for Schizophrenia and Other Common Mental Disorders,* 3d ed. (Eugene, OR: Borage Books, 2001): 143. G. Chouinard et al., "Tryptophan in the Treatment of Depression and Mania," *Advance in Biological Psychiatry* 10 (1983): 47–6. G. Chouinard et al., "A Controlled Clinical Trial of L-tryptophan in Acute Mania," *Biological Psychiatry* 20 (1985): 546–7.

113. "5-HTP, Omega-3 Acids Promising Treatments," *Autism Research Review International* 13:1 (1999): 2.

114. Eva Edelman, *Natural Healing,* 144.

115. Ronald Hoffman, "Beyond Prozac: Natural Therapies for Anxiety and Depression," *Innovation: The Health Letter of FAIM* (January 31, 1999): 10-11, 13, 15, 17, 19.

116. Linda Rector Page, N.D., Ph.D., *Healthy Healing: A Guide to Self-Healing for Everyone* (Carmel Valley, CA: Healthy Healing Publications, 1997): 103.

117. *DSM-IV-TR,* 478.

118. Michael Lesser, *Nutrition and Vitamin Therapy* (New York: Bantam, 1981):109–10.

119. Ronald Hoffman, "Beyond Prozac," 10–11, 13, 15, 17, 19.

120. Melvyn R. Werbach, M.D., *Nutritional Influences on Illness: A Sourcebook of Clinical Research* (Tarzana, CA: Third Line Press, 1994): 37–38. Michael Lesser, *Nutrition and Vitamin Therapy,* 109.

121. Ronald Hoffman, "Beyond Prozac," 10–11, 13, 15, 17, 19.

122. Ibid.

123. Michael Lesser, *Nutrition and Vitamin Therapy,* 73.

124. E. H. Cook and B. L. Leventhal, "The Serotonin System

in Autism," *Current Opinion in Pediatrics* 8:4 (August 1996): 348–54.

125. Syd Baumel, *Dealing with Depression Naturally*, 12.

126. National Alliance for the Mentally Ill (NAMI), "Obsessive-Compulsive Disorder," available on the Internet at: www.nami.org; or contact NAMI, Colonial Place Three, 2107 Wilson Blvd., Ste. 300, Alexandria, VA 22201-3042; tel: 888-999-NAMI (6264) or 703-524-7600.

127. NIH (National Institutes of Health), "Stress System Malfunction Could Lead to Serious, Life Threatening Disease," (September 9, 2002), article available on the Internet at: www.nichd.nih.gov/new/releases/stress.cfm.

128. Burton Goldberg and the editors of *Alternative Medicine, Alternative Medicine Women's Health Series: 2* (Tiburon, CA: Future Medicine Publishing, 1998): 208–209.

129. R. Reid, Wilson, Ph.D., *Don't Panic: Taking Control of Anxiety Attacks* (New York: HarperPerennial, 1996): 87.

130. Burton Goldberg and editors, *Alternative Medicine*, 21.

131. R. Reid Wilson, *Don't Panic*, 90–1.

132. Ibid., 104.

133. *DSM-IV-TR*, 481.

134. Ibid., 481. Harold H. Bloomfield, *Healing Anxiety Naturally*, 38.

135. Muriel MacFarlane, R.N., M.A., *The Panic Attack, Anxiety, and Phobia Solutions Handbook* (Leucadia, CA: United Research Publishers, 1995): 251-2.

136. Harold H. Bloomfield, *Healing Anxiety Naturally*, 40.

137. Jerilyn Ross, *Triumph Over Fear*, 265.

138. Eva Edelman, *Natural Healing*, 86.

139. Rita Elkins, *Depression and Natural Medicine: A Nutritional Approach to Depression and Mood Swings* (Pleasant Grove, UT: Woodland Publishing, 1995): 138.

140. Ibid.

141. Rita Elkins, *Depression and Natural Medicine*, 138. Eva Edelman, *Natural Healing*, 85.

142. Eva Edelman, *Natural Healing*, 84.

143. Ibid., 134.

144. Rita Elkins, *Depression and Natural Medicine,* 103. Eva Edelman, *Natural Healing,* 40.

145. Melvyn R. Werbach, M.D., *Nutritional Influences on Illness: A Sourcebook of Clinical Research* (Tarzana, CA: Third Line Press, 1994): 36.

146. Muriel MacFarlane, *Panic Attack Handbook,* 175-6.

147. A. Dunne, "Some Effect of the Quality of Light on Health," *Journal of Orthomolecular Medicine* 4:4 (1989): 229–32. John Nash Ott, *Health and Light* (Old Greenwich, CT: Devin-Adair, 1973).

148. David Kaiser, M.D., "Not by Chemicals Alone: A Hard Look at Psychiatric Medicine," *Psychiatric Times* 13:12 (Dec. 1996).

3: A Model for Healing

149. Simon Y. Mills, M.A., M.N.I.M.H., *The Dictionary of Modern Herbalism* (Rochester, VT: Healing Arts Press, 1988): 109.

150. NIMH, "Anxiety Disorders."

151. Richard Leviton, "Migraines, Seizures, and Mercury Toxicity," *Alternative Medicine Digest* 21 (December 1997/January 1998): 61.

4: Traditional Chinese Medicine

152. Shirley Babior and Carol Goldman, *Overcoming Panic, Anxiety, & Phobias: New Strategies to Free Yourself from Worry and Fear* (Duluth, MN: Whole Person Associates, 1996): 22.

5: Homeopathy

153. Judyth Reichenberg-Ullman, N.D., L.C.S.W., and Robert Ullman, N.D., *Prozac Free: Homeopathic Alternatives to Conventional Drug Therapies* (Berkeley, CA: North Atlantic Books, 2002): xiv.

154. Ibid.

155. Mary Ellin Lerner, "Facing Your Fear," *USA Weekend* (September 29–October 1, 2000): 9.

156. Miranda Castro, R.S.Hom., *The Complete Homeopathy Handbook* (New York: St. Martin's Press, 1991): 3–5. Anne Woodham and David Peters, M.D., *DK Encyclopedia of Healing Therapies* (New York: Dorling Kindersley, 1997): 126.

157. Judyth Reichenberg-Ullman, N.D., M.S.W., and Robert Ullman, N.D., *Ritalin-Free Kids: Safe and Effective Homeopathic*

Medicine for ADHD and Other Behavioral and Learning Problems (Roseville, CA: Prima Health, 2000): 95.

158. *Ritalin-Free Kids,* 95–96.

159. Personal communication and *Ritalin-Free Kids,* 90.

160. Personal communication and *Prozac Free,* 57.

161. *Ritalin-Free Kids,* 83.

162. Tinus Smits, "The Post-Vaccination Syndrome: Prevention," available on the Internet at www.tinussmits.com/english.

6: Flower Essence Therapy

163. Edward Bach and F. J. Wheeler, *The Bach Flower Remedies* (New Canaan, CT: Keats Publishing, 1977).

164. Patricia Kaminski and Richard Katz, *Flower Essence Repertory* (Nevada City, CA: Flower Essence Society, 1996): 5. Patricia Kaminski and Richard Katz, "Using Flower Essences: A Practical Overview," Nevada City, CA: Flower Essence Society, 1994.

165. Patricia Kaminski and Richard Katz, *Flower Essence Repertory,* 3.

166. "The Flower Essence Society: Pioneering Research and Education in Flower Essence Therapy," booklet published by the Flower Essence Society, Nevada City, CA: 10.

167. Jeffrey Cram, Ph.D., "FES Launches a Major Multi-Site Scientific Study on Flower Essences and the Treatment of Depression," *Flower Essence Society Newsletter* (Spring 2000): 1.

168. In a dissertation entitled "Continuing Education in Cuban Healthcare: Holistic Medicine and Flower Essence Therapy" for Florida State University, College of Education (Tallahassee, Fall 2002), Dr. Beatriz Miyar documented the training of 1,450 medical practitioners in Cuba (which took place in ten of Cuba's 15 provinces) as flower essence therapists in a program sponsored by the Cuban Ministry of Public Health. In a personal communication with the author (2003), Dr. Miyar summarized her findings: "In seeking solutions to help their patients receive better quality of care, motivated and committed health professionals in Cuba began treating their patients with FET with encouraging and positive results, including increased patient demand. When it became obvious that FET is free of harmful side effects, simple to practice, and with no significant budgetary

demands, the Ministry of Public Health officially recognized it as a valid medical modality. . . . There is no other country in the world that has medical professionals and patient population as knowledgeable in flower essence therapy as is currently the case in Cuba. Continuing professional education, both formal and informal, has played an absolutely central role in the development of this phenomenon."

7: Soma Therapies

169. Alice Quaid, P.T., "Post-Traumatic Stress Disorder: Veterans and Other Patients Find Hope Through Body-Mind Therapies," *PT & OT Today* (January 20, 1997); available at the Upledger Institute website: www.upledger.com/news/9701a.htm.

170. Richard Leviton, "Reversing Autism and Depression with Bodywork," *Alternative Medicine* 24 (June/July 1998): 36–41.

171. "CranioSacral Therapy," available at the Upledger Institute website (www.upledger.com/therapies/cst.htm).

172. "What Is Osteopathy?" available at the Cranial Academy website (www.cranialacademy.org/whatis.html).

173. "CranioSacral Therapy," available at the Upledger Institute website (www.upledger.com/therapies/cst.htm).

174. Sources: Informational materials of Soma Therapy Centres; and Richard Leviton, "Reversing Autism and Depression with Bodywork," 36–41.

8: Thought Field Therapy and Seemorg Matrix Work

175. Roger J. Callahan, Ph.D., *The Anxiety-Addiction Connection: Eliminate Your Addictive Urges with Thought Field Therapy* (Indian Wells, CA: Roger J. Callahan, Ph.D., 1995): 5. Available from: The Callahan Techniques, La Quinta, CA; 760-564–1008.

176. Roger J. Callahan, Ph.D., *Tapping the Healer Within: Using Thought Field Therapy to Instantly Conquer Your Fears, Anxieties, and Emotional Distress* (Chicago: Contemporary Books, 2001): 12.

177. Ibid., 47.

178. Raeann Dumont, *The Sky Is Falling: Understanding and Coping with Phobias, Panic, and Obsessive-Compulsive Disorders* (New York: W.W. Norton, 1996): 214–5.

179. Nahoma Asha Clinton, L.C.S.W., Ph.D., "Seemorg Matrix Work, The Transpersonal Energy Psychotherapy," available on the Internet at www.matrixwork.org/tara.html.

180. Ibid.

181. Nahoma Asha Clinton, L.C.S.W., Ph.D., "The Story of SEEMORG," available on the Internet at www.seemorgmatrix.org/seemorg-story.html.

182. Nahoma Asha Clinton, L.C.S.W., Ph.D., "Redefining Trauma," available on the Internet at www.matrixwork.org/manual.htm.

9: Psychic and Shamanic Healing

183. Richard Leviton, *The Healthy Living Space* (Charlottesville, VA: Hampton Roads, 2001): 354–8.

184. Ibid., 362–3.

185. Ibid., 364.

186. John Lash, *The Seeker's Handbook* (New York: Harmony Books, 1990): 371.

187. Muriel MacFarlane, R.N., M.A., *The Panic Attack, Anxiety, and Phobia Solutions Handbook* (Leucadia, CA: United Research Publishers, 1995): 60.

188. Malidoma Patrice Somé, *Ritual: Power, Healing, and Community* (New York: Penguin, 1997): 12, 19.

189. Malidoma Patrice Somé, *Of Water and the Spirit: Ritual, Magic, and Initiation in the Life of an African Shaman* (New York: Penguin, 1994): 9, 10.

Index

About the Author

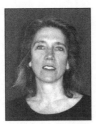 Stephanie Marohn has been writing since she was a child. Her adult writing background is extensive in both journalism and nonfiction trade books. In addition to *Natural Medicine First Aid Remedies* and the six books in the Healthy Mind series (*The Natural Medicine Guide to Autism, The Natural Medicine Guide to Depression, The Natural Medicine Guide to Bipolar Disorder, The Natural Medicine Guide to Addiction, The Natural Medicine Guide to Anxiety,* and *The Natural Medicine Guide to Schizophrenia*), she has published more than thirty articles in magazines and newspapers, written two novels and a feature film screenplay, and has had her work included in poetry, prayer, and travel writing anthologies.

Originally from Philadelphia, she has been a resident of the San Francisco Bay Area for over twenty years, and currently lives in Sonoma County, north of the city.

Please visit www.stephaniemarohn.com for more information.

Hampton Roads Publishing Company

... for the evolving human spirit

Hampton Roads Publishing Company
publishes books on a variety of subjects,
including metaphysics, health,
visionary fiction, and other related topics.

For a copy of our latest catalog, call toll-free
(800) 766-8009, or send your name and address to:

Hampton Roads Publishing Company, Inc.
1125 Stoney Ridge Road
Charlottesville, VA 22902

e-mail: hrpc@hrpub.com
www.hrpub.com